Balanced Ethics Review

Simon N. Whitney

Balanced Ethics Review

A Guide for Institutional Review
Board Members

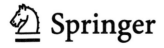 Springer

Simon N. Whitney, MD, JD
Associate Professor and William O'Donnell
    and Regina O'Donnell Chair
    in Family Medicine
Department of Family and
    Community Medicine
Associate Professor, Center for Medical
    Ethics and Health Policy
Baylor College of Medicine
Houston, TX, USA

ISBN 978-3-319-20704-9   ISBN 978-3-319-20705-6 (eBook)
DOI 10.1007/978-3-319-20705-6
Springer Cham Heidelberg New York Dordrecht London

Library of Congress Control Number: 2015946614

Printed on acid-free paper

Springer International Publishing AG Switzerland is part of Springer Science+Business Media (www.springer.com)

With gratitude to:
Patricia Serventi Naughton
Eunice Thomas

Preface

This manual will help you, the IRB member or chair, conduct ethics review that balances the two major moral considerations in research with human subjects.

Balance

This guide would not have been needed when the IRB system was formed, for ethical pioneers like Hans Jonas, Paul Ramsey, and Henry Beecher took balance for granted. They recognized that research ethics should aim to promote both the rights and welfare of research subjects and our shared interest in better treatments for disease. In the past half century, however, theory and practice have turned away from the balanced perspective of the early ethicists and toward an exclusive focus on subject protection.

Today's error has virtuous roots. Scholars in the mid-twentieth century were drawn to research ethics by grievously unethical experiments like the Tuskegee syphilis study and the Jewish Chronic Disease Hospital cancer cell injections. Early ethicists focused on protecting subjects from serious hazards. When study subjects risked death, any benefit to society was rightly dismissed as unimportant.

Once the foundations were laid—once the moral contours of injury and abuse were charted and a regulatory system established to guard against those perils—later ethicists turned to lesser risks, ultimately creating a literature that paid increasing attention to diminishing hazards.

The result is today's unbalanced ethics, in which the benefits research brings to society are discounted as morally irrelevant.

This manual will give you the tools to restore the balance that the early ethicists saw as fundamental.

The Curse of Power

Many contemporary IRBs have lost both balance and focus. The system was created to protect subjects, but IRBs today sometimes seek to protect scientists, to forestall controversy, to prevent lawsuits, and to improve the methodology of the science they review. These activities are all manifestations of the curse of power—the belief that the IRB has an open-ended mandate to take any action that would improve the research enterprise. IRBs should shun these distractions and focus on protecting subjects.

Changing Ethics and Unchanging Regulation

Ethical principles may be universal, but ethical practice is contextual. Early scholarship assumed, for instance, that enrollment in a randomized trial jeopardized subjects' welfare and was therefore morally questionable. This assumption was overturned when patients with AIDS demanded inclusion in trials of new drugs. The realization that trial participation can be a benefit does not displace our older concern about participation as a burden; each is valid in the appropriate circumstance.

New research methods expose deficiencies in the ethical canon. The Nuremberg Code states unconditionally that the consent of the subject is essential, but a stubborn insistence on consent can make research less ethical. We must question fixed principles that arise from archetypal abuses and embrace the new and more nuanced morality that leading scholars now propose.

This new morality overruns the bounds of today's regulatory structure. The regulations might be interpreted in a way that permits IRBs to follow contemporary ethical theory, but creative ethical solutions are not welcomed by the federal oversight agencies. This manual candidly explains when federal policy restricts your IRB's ability to adapt to our changing scientific and moral landscape.

Still there is much to celebrate. Ethicists find new ways to help science; science finds new ways to help us all. Your IRB will play an important role in these advances.

This manual focuses on ethics review in the USA. But the challenges of ethics review are international, so I hope that it may be of some use in other countries that recognize that subjects and society both matter.

About this Manual

This guide is filled with the insights of dozens of scholars. If you want to learn more about any topic in this manual, start with the references. I host a website, http://balancedethicsreview.com, and invite you to participate in the ongoing discussion there.

No guide can provide the final answer for ethical uncertainty. This manual covers some core issues but omits others, such as proxy consent to research, research with prisoners, research with children, and placebo-controlled trials; it considers federal, but not state or local, regulations. And because it focuses on ethics, not procedures, this manual omits the mechanical details of IRB operations like how many members a committee must have and what kinds of research qualify for exempt or expedited review; your IRB chair or administrator will guide you in these matters. Robert Amdur and Elizabeth Bankert's *Institutional Review Board Member Handbook* (2011c) provides an excellent discussion of how an effective IRB functions.

I mention individual authors when there are one or two; in the interests of readability, when there are three or more I sometimes mention only the first author and dispense with the customary but cumbersome "*et al*" or "and colleagues."

The people who make research possible are commonly referred to as "subjects," although some authors believe it is more respectful to refer to them as "participants." I follow the more common usage of "subject" while applauding the individuals who, far from being passive objects of study, are active partners in the research.

This guide has benefited from candid review by my friends, family, and colleagues, and it is as accurate and sensible as I know how to make it, but I do not imagine that it is without error or beyond improvement. If you have comments or criticisms, please email me at swhitney@bcm.edu.

Where to Start Reading

This manual is meant to be useful to the IRB member at any level of experience. Chapter 1 summarizes the entire guide. The remainder of the book provides the reasoning, authorities, arguments, and counterarguments.

If you are contemplating joining the IRB but have not yet done so, be advised that the IRB is like no other committee. It deals with issues of vital importance to your university, medical school, or hospital, and it may require correspondingly outsize effort from you. Please read Sect. 2.6, "Your IRB Service," which reviews the terms of your IRB service.

If you are a new IRB member I suggest you begin with Chap. 1, the Introduction, which includes a compact summary of the book and the essential ethical concepts any member needs to know.

If you are a community member, please see especially Sect. 2.6.3, "The Community Member."

If your IRB is dedicated to research in the social sciences, Chap. 6 is for you. Browsing through Chap. 1 will help you find additional relevant material.

If you are an experienced IRB member or chair, you can start with Chap. 1 for a rapid overview, or Chap. 2, which begins the detailed discussion of ethics review.

Houston, TX, USA   Simon N. Whitney

Acknowledgements

This book has benefited from thoughtful critiques by many people. Eunice Thomas read the manuscript with a care and skill that reflect decades of experience as an attorney and judge, and then provided me with the candid feedback that only a sibling could provide. My daughter, Diana Whitney, helped me reach an appropriately collegial tone. Judy Levison, my ex-wife, has provided encouragement and counsel for years.

Patricia Serventi Naughton found innumerable tactful ways to bring me closer to the truth on key issues, including the relationship between ethics and regulation.

Regina O'Donnell, by endowing the William O'Donnell and Regina O'Donnell Chair in Family Medicine, gave me time, any scholar's most precious resource.

Jon Tyson, director of the Center for Clinical Research and Evidence Based Medicine at the University of Texas Health Science Center at Houston, provided funding. Michelle Smith, the Center's administrator, coordinated meetings in which Jon, Paula Knudson, Susan Wootton, Patricia Evans, and Kathleen Kennedy shared with me their views and experiences.

Carl E. Schneider, during 6 years of close collaboration, shared with me his extraordinary insights into law and society. Shawna Peterson, Sarah Glass, and Jennifer Pratt Mead have given encouragement and support. Barbara Evans, Emil Freireich, Daniel Musher, Pauline Rosenau, Vance Hamilton, and Razelle Kurzrock have shared ideas and comments. I am honored to have the assistance of such distinguished people.

I am grateful for the academic and administrative support of Roger Zoorob, Sara Rahman, Stephen Spann, Robert Volk, and Atma Ram of the Department of Family and Community Medicine at Baylor College of Medicine. My family medicine colleagues David Buck, Jason Salemi, and Hamisu Salihu have given their advice freely.

Amy McGuire and the other members of the Baylor College of Medicine Center for Medical Ethics and Health Policy discussed sections of this manual during our journal club and provided helpful suggestions. Larry McCullough, channeling Leibniz over lunch, advised me to consider Springer as a publisher. Brenda Hart, Baylor's HIPAA specialist, shared her expertise.

Mats Hansson and Pär Segerdahl have welcomed me on my visits to Sweden and provided a vital international perspective.

I got my start in human subjects protection at Stanford in 1995–1999, where I was fortunate to work with Hank Greeley of the Law School, Tom Raffin and Ernlé Young, codirectors of the Stanford Center for Biomedical Ethics, and Donna Adelman and the outstanding members and staff of the Stanford IRB. Ernlé read a draft of this manual in 2014 and pointed out that the typical new IRB member is going to want a low calorie option; the introductory chapter is the fruit of this sensible observation. Joan Rachlin, by inviting me to speak at the 2007 PRIM&R conference, helped me reconnect with working IRB members and administrators.

Authors need help from publishing experts. Jane Isay, a friend since my Yale Press days (when we edited with pencils) helped me navigate the byways of contemporary publishing. Elizabeth Knoll of Harvard University Press helped with a related book, one that made this manual possible. Susan Hatch, of Oxford Editing, arranged for Jennifer Keane to double-check every citation—a great comfort for the anxious author of a book that draws on 199 sources.

The Springer team, including Greg Sutorius, Portia Wong, and Richard Lansing, has been a pleasure to work with. I appreciate the careful copy editing of Sathiyaraj N and the hard work of project manager Vijay Shanker. My work at Yale Press left me with one understanding of how a manuscript should become a book. Springer has shown me another way, one that gives the author more control over content and fewer worries about design. Thanks to Springer's efficient process, the first signed copy will be in the hands of my son, Jordan Whitney, half a year sooner than it would be with a traditional publisher.

Contents

1   **Introduction**   1
    1.1   Overview   1
    1.2   Ethics and the IRB   1
    1.3   IRB Process...   3
    1.4   Evaluating Biomedical Research   4
    1.5   Consent in Biomedical Research   5
    1.6   The Social Sciences   6
    1.7   Biomedical Research Topics.....................................   7
    1.8   FDA and OHRP   10
    1.9   The Future...   10

2   **Ethics and the IRB**...   11
    2.1   Your Influential Position   11
    2.2   Evidence..   12
    2.3   Scandal   12
    2.4   Research Ethics...   13
        2.4.1   Two Ethical Principles   13
        2.4.2   Two Ethical Goals..   14
        2.4.3   Goals into Practice   14
        2.4.4   Today's Loss of Balance   15
        2.4.5   It's Always About People..............................   16
    2.5   Ethical Goals and Regulatory Means........................   17
        2.5.1   Principles of Regulation................................   17
        2.5.2   Organization and Legal Framework   18
    2.6   Your IRB Service   18
        2.6.1   Compensation   19

2.6.2 Protection from Lawsuits 19
2.6.3 The Community Member 20
2.7 The Triumph of Ethics Review 21
3 IRB Process 23
3.1 Principles 23
3.1.1 Respectfulness 23
3.1.2 Transparency 24
3.1.3 Efficiency 25
3.1.4 Clarity 25
3.1.5 Accountability 26
3.1.6 Judiciousness 26
3.1.7 Rationality 27
3.1.8 Restraint 27
3.2 The Curse of Power 27
3.2.1 Scope of IRB Authority 28
3.2.2 Litigation Prevention 29
3.2.3 Beyond the Regulations 30
4 Evaluating Biomedical Research 33
4.1 The Objective IRB 33
4.1.1 Ramsey and the Scientist's Bias 33
4.1.2 Your Reasonable Understanding 34
4.2 Literature Reviews 35
4.2.1 Death at Johns Hopkins 35
4.2.2 Reviews by Investigators 35
4.2.3 Reviews by IRBs 36
4.3 Ethics and Science 36
4.3.1 Scientific Modifications 37
4.3.2 The Value of Research 37
4.3.3 Risk 38
4.4 Weighing Risks, Benefits, and Knowledge 39
4.4.1 Why You Should Protect Subjects 40
4.4.2 Why You Should Let Subjects Choose 41
4.4.3 The Conundrum 42
4.5 Approval Based on Risk and Benefit 42
4.5.1 Established Theories 43
4.5.2 Rajczi and Meyer: Let the Subjects Decide 44
4.6 Consent Before Approval 45

5   Consent in Biomedical Research   47
   5.1   Consent's Goals   47
   5.2   Multisite Consent Forms   47
   5.3   Presenting Risk and Benefit   48
   5.4   Subject Understanding   50
         5.4.1   Less Is More   50
         5.4.2   Ethical Considerations   51
   5.5   Supervising Consent Form Writing   52
         5.5.1   Helping the Investigator   52
         5.5.2   Readability   53
         5.5.3   Format   53
   5.6   Editing the Consent Form   55

6   The Social Sciences   57
   6.1   The Value of Dissent   57
   6.2   The Social Impact of Research   58
   6.3   Freedom of Speech   59
   6.4   Psychology   60
         6.4.1   Deception   61
         6.4.2   Threats to Self-Esteem   61
   6.5   Surveys and Interviews   63
         6.5.1   Risk and Benefit   63
         6.5.2   Modifications   65
   6.6   Field Research   65
         6.6.1   Risk   65
         6.6.2   The Sociologists' Dispute   66
   6.7   Racial Discrimination   68

7   Biomedical Research Topics   71
   7.1   Archival Research   71
         7.1.1   Cancer of the Vagina   71
         7.1.2   Regulatory Oversight   72
         7.1.3   Ethical Considerations   73
         7.1.4   The Common Rule   74
         7.1.5   HIPAA   75
   7.2   The Learning Health Care System   78
         7.2.1   Integrating Research and Clinical Care   78
         7.2.2   Ethical Considerations   79
         7.2.3   Your IRB's Role   80

7.3   Randomized Controlled Trials 80
       7.3.1   Risks Inside and Outside of a Trial 81
       7.3.2   Nonphysical Risks 82
7.4   Comparative Effectiveness Trials 83
       7.4.1   Identifying the Better Treatment 83
       7.4.2   Faden's Bold Ethical Proposal 84
       7.4.3   Waiver of Consent in Special
               Circumstances 85
7.5   Justice 86
       7.5.1   Unjust Burdens 86
       7.5.2   The Governmental Pursuit of Justice 87
       7.5.3   The Private Pursuit of Justice 88
7.6   The Vulnerable 88
       7.6.1   Regulatory Overprotection 88
       7.6.2   Fighting Health Disparities 89
7.7   Paying Subjects 90
       7.7.1   Respecting Subject Choice 91
       7.7.2   Coercion 92
       7.7.3   Setting a Cap on Wages 93
7.8   Emergency Research 93
       7.8.1   Criteria for Approval 94
       7.8.2   Ethical Considerations 95
7.9   Phase 1 Cancer Trials 96

8 FDA and OHRP 99
8.1   Agencies Under Pressure 99
8.2   Your IRB and the Agencies 100
       8.2.1   Balancing Three Goals 101
       8.2.2   When Regulations Trump Ethics 101
       8.2.3   The Successful IRB 102
       8.2.4   Things Can Go Wrong 103
8.3   Pushing Back Against Federal Pressure 103
       8.3.1   The Agency 103
       8.3.2   The Funder 104
       8.3.3   The Media 105
       8.3.4   The Courts 106
8.4   Risk and Your IRB 106

9 The Future 107
   9.1 Evidence 107
   9.2 Reform 108
   9.3 The Challenge 110

References 111

Index 123

Chapter 1
Introduction

1.1 Overview

The manual is summarized in this introductory chapter. This chapter's contents are largely omitted from the index; instead, the chapter is keyed so that you can easily turn to the appropriate section later in the book. It includes the critical questions that your Institutional Review Board (IRB) should consider as you conduct ethics review. The analyses, differing points of view, and names and citations are provided in later chapters, so if you want the details, begin with Chap. 2. Otherwise this introduction is the place to start.

1.2 Ethics and the IRB

Your Influential Position. IRB permission is required for most research with people, including research regulated by the Food and Drug Administration (FDA) or funded by the National Institutes of Health (NIH). Typically, the scientist or scholar submits a proposal; the IRB approves it, rejects it, or returns it with instructions for changes. Most IRBs are situated in hospitals, government agencies, or institutions of learning (including universities, medical schools, and research institutes); the rest are independent, either nonprofit or for profit. All follow the same rules (see Sect. 2.1).

© Springer International Publishing Switzerland 2016
S.N. Whitney, *Balanced Ethics Review*,
DOI 10.1007/978-3-319-20705-6_1

Evidence. Your IRB should draw on evidence whenever possible. There is no reason to speculate when we have data (see Sect. 2.2).

Scandal. The IRB system was created in response to unethical research conducted in the mid-twentieth century. The most infamous was the Tuskegee syphilis study, in which government doctors actively kept poor black sharecroppers with the disease from obtaining treatment (see Sect. 2.3).

Research Ethics. Henry Beecher was among the first to expose unethical experimentation; other early ethicists have had an enduring influence as well. The Belmont Report, the most influential document in the field, analyzes research ethics in terms of the moral principles of beneficence (concern for the welfare of others), respect for persons (concern for the rights of others), and justice (see Sect. 2.4).

Two Ethical Principles. This manual rests on two ethical principles. As responsible people, we have (at least) two obligations:
• Do no harm to others, and
• Help others (see Sect. 2.4.1).

Two Ethical Goals. The two principles translate directly into your IRB's two ethical goals—to protect subjects and to enable research that will benefit society. Research ethics has traditionally focused on protecting human subjects from injury ("do no harm"), but that is only one piece of the picture. The other ethical centerpiece is the role of scholarly and scientific investigation in improving our health and our society ("help others"). It is, for instance, highly ethical to conduct research that reduces the burden of cancer, lessens the disparities in health between rich and poor, or exposes racial discrimination (see Sect. 2.4.2).

Today's Loss of Balance. Some authors have become persuaded that IRBs should be concerned only with subject safety. This was not the intention of the system's founders, who meant the system to both protect subjects and make possible research that benefits the public. Your IRB should consider both the subject and society (see Sect. 2.4.4).

It's Always About People. For your IRB, science matters because it helps people. The scientists and scholars that you supervise deserve fair treatment, but your moral focus is on the ordinary people, unknown and perhaps unborn, whose health and lives will benefit (see Sect. 2.4.5).

Ethical Goals and Regulatory Means. Your IRB's decisions should be respected because they are ethically persuasive; they must be obeyed because you hold federal power. You pursue ethical goals through regulatory means (see Sect. 2.5).

Your IRB Service. Work on the IRB can be demanding. You should serve on equitable terms, fairly compensated and adequately protected. If you are the community member, you can serve in any way that makes sense to you and your IRB chair (see Sect. 2.6).

The Triumph of Ethics Review. The IRB system, exported in 1966 from the NIH to every research-oriented institution, dramatically reduced unethical experimentation. This is the triumph of ethics review. It is an important contribution to society, and I hope it is one of the reasons you are willing to serve on the IRB (see Sect. 2.7).

1.3   IRB Process

Principles. Proper procedures facilitate wise decisions. Your IRB should honor the virtues of:
- Respectfulness, treating investigators as valued colleagues (see Sect. 3.1.1)
- Transparency, with your operations open to public view (see Sect. 3.1.2)
- Efficiency, minimizing the cost of your review in time and money (see Sect. 3.1.3)
- Clarity, using language in appropriate ways (see Sect. 3.1.4)
- Accountability, providing an appeals process (see Sect. 3.1.5)
- Judiciousness, acting only when the benefits justify the costs (see Sect. 3.1.6)
- Rationality, striving to improve the public interest in ways that are evidence-based (see Sect. 3.1.7)
- Restraint, remaining within the bounds of your authority (see Sect. 3.1.8)

The Curse of Power. Your IRB has dominion over dozens or hundreds of scientists and scholars; you approve or reject hundreds or thousands of requests annually. You were given this power to protect the rights and welfare of subjects, but the regulations do not say that you must restrict your attention to this goal. Because your committee has plenary power over research with humans, well-meaning people will attempt to hijack you to serve their purposes (see Sect. 3.2). Your IRB should resist when others encourage you to:

- Protect anyone or anything except research subjects (you are not responsible for the welfare of the investigator, for instance; see Sect. 3.2.1)
- Protect your institution from litigation (it has other defenses; see Sect. 3.2.2)
- Go beyond the regulations, imposing additional burdens on research (see Sect. 3.2.3).

1.4   Evaluating Biomedical Research

The Objective IRB. Although your committee has scientists, it is unlikely to understand any given study as well as the investigators who wrote it. This is not a defect; it is an inherent feature of IRB review, and your distance is an asset as you evaluate a protocol's ethics. You are not reviewing protocols because you are more ethical than the researchers, but because you are more objective (see Sect. 4.1).

Literature Reviews. Scientists need to be in command of their fields. Some IRBs therefore require the investigator to submit a review of the literature with each application. This requirement goes beyond what the regulations demand—an example of the curse of power. There is also no evidence that this practice improves subject protection (see Sect. 4.2).

Scientific Modifications. Some IRBs are charged by the institution with critiquing the methodology of protocols. If your IRB is not intended to serve in a scientific advisory capacity—if your only mission is to conduct ethics review—you should not modify the science of the protocols you review (see Sect. 4.3.1).

The Value of Research. Your IRB has the authority to reject a proposal when you believe it has no value, particularly if it exposes subjects to risk, but you should do so with care (see Sect. 4.3.2).

Weighing Risks, Benefits, and Knowledge. The regulations require
your IRB to approve only protocols whose risks are justified by the
study's benefits and the knowledge the study is expected to produce. It
can be difficult to decide how risky a protocol you can approve. As you
weigh a protocol's risks, benefits, and promised knowledge, two of the
Belmont Report principles urge you in opposite directions. Beneficence
(concern for another's welfare) instructs you to protect prospective
subjects from risks that you feel are excessive. Respect for persons
encourages you to allow subjects to decide, based on the risks as they
see them. This is a quandary with no easy answer (see Sect. 4.4).

Approval Based on Risk and Benefit. There are several theories about
how your IRB can decide when research is too risky to permit; none has
been thoroughly tested in actual committee operations (see Sect. 4.5).

Consent Before Approval. One novel way your IRB might approach
this problem is by giving the investigator permission to discuss the
research with prospective subjects and obtain their consent, but not to
begin the actual research. You could then meet with some of these
people to learn more about their understanding of the risks and benefits of the research. Ultimately you would either permit the protocol
to begin or decide that the subjects are not making an informed and
voluntary decision (see Sect. 4.6).

1.5   Consent in Biomedical Research

Consent's Goals. Consent enables subjects to enroll in research on
their own terms and makes possible research that will benefit us all.
Consent does *not* to funnel more subjects into research; it helps each
person make the choice that is right for him or her (see Sect. 5.1).

Multisite Consent Forms. Your IRB should not alter the consent
forms of protocols from outside your institution (see Sect. 5.2).

Presenting Risk and Benefit. For protocols from your institution, your
IRB should ensure that the consent form presents the study's risks
and benefits as accurately as possible. It should neither highlight a
study's benefits and downplay its risks, nor exaggerate risks and
understate benefits; either deprives prospective subjects of information they need (see Sect. 5.3).

Subject Understanding. Potential subjects decide whether to partici-pate in a study based on their knowledge of it, so the more they understand, the better. Ideally, subjects will become so familiar with the proposed research that their decision reflects their individual val-ues and preferences. Your IRB should help prospective subjects understand research as well as they can; but no matter how clearly information is provided, not every subject wants to be, or can be, accurately and thoroughly informed. Accordingly, investigators must disclose information, but subjects do not have to fully comprehend that information for their consent to be valid (see Sect. 5.4).

Supervising Consent Form Writing. You should try to provide such clear instructions that local investigators write forms that you can approve without changing a word. You should consider formatting the consent form so that the most important information, presented in the simplest possible language, appears first, followed by material that is less central to subject understanding. An ideal consent form has a minimum of material that is irrelevant or foolish (see Sect. 5.5).

Editing the Consent Form. Edit consent forms only when there is a serious problem (see Sect. 5.6).

1.6   The Social Sciences

The Value of Dissent. If your IRB reviews research in the social sci-ences, you will have a ringside seat as scholars study such sensitive issues as racial and gender discrimination. You should interfere only when there is risk to subjects. You have a duty to approve research that will help ground public debate in evidence (see Sect. 6.1).

The Social Impact of Research. Your IRB might be tempted to hinder research whose results might support a particular political viewpoint about gun control, discrimination, or other charged topics. The regu-lations, however, advise you not to block protocols based on your fear that they might lead to socially undesirable results. You are respon-sible for the risks to subjects, not to society (see Sect. 6.2).

Freedom of Speech. Is it censorship when an IRB at a state university interferes with survey or interview research? Some legal experts feel it is; others do not. You can stay clear of this controversy by permitting scholars to conduct survey and interview research even if you believe the questions, or the study's goals, are immoral or antisocial (see Sect. 6.3).

Psychology. Psychologists routinely conduct research that involves deception; proper practice requires that subjects be debriefed afterward. Even experiments that shake subjects' self-esteem may be ethical with proper safeguards (see Sect. 6.4).

Surveys and Interviews. Your IRB is likely to review many survey and interview studies, whose chief hazard is the inadvertent redisclosure of information; you should therefore make sure that confidential data are secure. Other risks seldom merit attention. The evidence indicates that responding to questions, even on sensitive topics, is rarely hazardous enough to warrant your intervention (see Sect. 6.5).

Field Research. Some social scientists study people and communities by observing or participating in their activities. There is controversy within the discipline as to whether these scholars should disclose their identity and obtain consent, but unless an investigation threatens to harm individuals there is no reason for your IRB to interfere (see Sect. 6.6).

Racial Discrimination. Some social scientists study discrimination by sending matched pairs of testers (e.g., one white and one minority) to apply for housing or employment. Studies using this well-respected method are presumptively ethical (see Sect. 6.7).

1.7 Biomedical Research Topics

Archival Research. Routine medical care generates copious amounts of data and specimens. Investigators can study this material by using it in deidentified form or by obtaining consent from individual patients; when neither of those approaches is feasible, your IRB may be asked to authorize its use without consent. In general, you may waive the requirement for consent if the research could not practicably be conducted without the waiver (see Sect. 7.1).

The Learning Health Care System. Ordinary clinical care and medical research, which were once distinct, are increasingly being combined on a large scale. The records from medical practice will soon be routinely used for research, and the results of the research be used to improve clinical practice; this combination of research and practice is called the learning health care system. Some ethicists believe that patients have an obligation to allow their data to be used in this system, but the regulations do not, so far, allow this (see Sect. 7.2).

Randomized Controlled Trials. By analyzing mountains of data, the learning health care system can show, for instance, a strong correlation between a particular treatment and lower mortality. But simply observing the outcomes of different patients given different treatments does not prove causality. When scientists want to prove that an intervention saves lives, a randomized controlled trial is usually best. Some randomized trials pose thorny ethical issues or present unusual hazards, but for a typical study, subjects in the trial will fare about as well as patients given routine care outside it (see Sect. 7.3).

Comparative Effectiveness Trials. A comparative effectiveness trial is a special type of randomized trial in which both interventions are already in routine clinical use. By definition, it poses no risks beyond those of ordinary clinical care. Some ethicists believe that, in a clinic or hospital that is operated with transparency and the active involvement of patients, subjects should not have to give consent to be enrolled in some kinds of comparative effectiveness trials. Federal agencies nonetheless require comprehensive consent (see Sect. 7.4).

Justice. It offends justice when one group reaps the benefit of research while another bears its burdens. Today, some research is specifically designed to decrease health disparities, and poor people who enroll in research are often paid. But injustices remain important even though they are less common. Your IRB should act when it identifies a problematic distribution of burdens and benefits (see Sect. 7.5.1).

The Governmental Pursuit of Justice. Congress, with executive branch input, provides funding that prioritizes research in diseases that inflict the greatest burden of suffering and in critical problems like racial health disparities; senior federal officials implement these priorities as they allocate funds to thousands of specific projects. Your IRB promotes justice every time it approves a protocol that is part of this comprehensive program. You should not modify or disapprove individual protocols in an attempt to serve justice unless you are unusually well-informed about the overall federal plan (see Sect. 7.5.2).

The Private Pursuit of Justice. IRBs review research funded by pharmaceutical companies and nonprofit groups like the American Heart Association. Your IRB should not modify or block these protocols in an attempt to promote justice (see Sect. 7.5.3).

The Vulnerable. Some groups, such as children, prisoners, and mentally disabled persons, are handicapped in their efforts to seize opportunity and avoid peril. For the vulnerable, as for us all, sound ethics balances risk and benefit. Your IRB should prevent the vulnerable from being conscripted for harmful research; it should also permit the vulnerable to participate in research in which some well-informed subjects might want to join. Your IRB helps reduce health disparities when it ensures that vulnerable subjects are enrolled in appropriate research (see Sect. 7.6).

Paying Subjects. People enroll in research to get better care, to help others, to be paid, and for other reasons; none is morally suspect and none should attract undue IRB attention. If a subject who has been properly informed wants to get better care, to help others, or to make money, that is not an ethical predicament; it is how people make decisions. The IRB should usually permit scientists to offer more money to persuade more prospective subjects to enroll (see Sect. 7.7).

Emergency Research. If we are to conduct research in emergency conditions at all, it must be without consent; and since the intervention being tested must offer the prospect of direct benefit, the waiver of consent is ethically sound. Your IRB may therefore approve research in emergency medical conditions if the regulatory requirements are met (see Sect. 7.8).

Phase 1 Cancer Trials. When animal research suggests that a new anticancer agent has promise, it is cautiously tested in small phase 1 trials, so named because they are the first phase of drug evaluation in humans. Patients are eligible only if they have failed any conventional therapy and are expected to die. Phase 1 trials offer a modest chance of benefit; they also provide a measure of hope to patients who have no other options. Phase 1 trial consent forms should not overstate the chance of benefit, but they need not attempt to crush hope (see Sect. 7.9).

1.8   FDA and OHRP

Agencies Under Pressure. The FDA and the Office for Human Research Protections (OHRP) supervise IRBs. Both agencies are positioned to improve the health and well-being of the American people. Unfortunately, like most federal bureaus, they are more often criticized for error than for inaction; this drives both agencies toward extremes of caution (see Sect. 8.1).

Your IRB and the Agencies. In 1998–2001, the FDA and OHRP temporarily shut down federally funded research at a dozen major institutions. In response, both affected and unaffected institutions showered new money and manpower on their IRBs. These well-supported committees were in no doubt that government sanctions must be avoided at all costs. The burst of disciplinary actions is over, but the threat remains. Your IRB must do its best to protect your institution from federal punishment (see Sect. 8.2).

Pushing Back Against Federal Pressure. If your IRB is under federal attack, you can resist through the media, the funder, or the courts (see Sect. 8.3).

Risk and Your IRB. Your IRB should not take careless chances, but if you seek perfect safety you will impose unconscionable costs on the research you supervise. Your IRB must itself accept a modicum of risk (see Sect. 8.4).

1.9   The Future

Evidence. Your IRB should use evidence whenever possible. I encourage you to also contribute to our knowledge about optimal IRB functioning (see Sect. 9.1).

Reform. Reform is badly needed, at every level from institutional policy to federal law (see Sect. 9.2).

The Challenge. Your IRB's task is complex. But if you follow sound ethical and regulatory principles, use your experience, and trust your common sense, you will succeed (see Sect. 9.3).

Chapter 2
Ethics and the IRB

You're on the Institutional Review Board. Congratulations!

2.1 Your Influential Position

IRB permission is required for most research with people, including research regulated by the FDA or funded by the NIH. Typically, the scientist or scholar submits a proposal; the IRB approves it, rejects it, or returns it with instructions for changes. Most IRBs are situated in hospitals, government agencies, and institutions of learning (including universities, medical schools, and research institutes); the rest are independent, either nonprofit or for profit. All follow the same rules.

This manual shows how to apply ethics in the daily operations of your IRB. It addresses the issues and dilemmas you will face as an IRB member and articulates the competing considerations you will need to balance. I host a website about ethics review at http://balancedethicsreview.com and invite you to join the conversation there.

If you are new to the IRB, you should give careful thought to the conditions of your service (see Sect. 2.6). If you are a community member, please see especially Sect. 2.6.3.

Your seat on the IRB puts you in a pivotal position in deciding what research will be permitted. You will review the ethics of research from academic niches in every corner of your university or medical school. Some new IRB members worry that they will be

© Springer International Publishing Switzerland 2016
S.N. Whitney, *Balanced Ethics Review*,
DOI 10.1007/978-3-319-20705-6_2

unequal to this responsibility, but not be intimidated. You don't need a doctorate in theoretical ethics. You need only learn the basics of practical ethics and regulation, and apply the relevant evidence.

2.2   Evidence

If ethics seems like an abstract field, you will be relieved to learn that your committee's deliberations are supported by a substantial body of evidence. Should you protect subjects from a survey about an upsetting experience? You don't have to guess—others have done the research to answer that question (see Sect. 6.5). How much do people sacrifice when they enroll in a typical randomized trial? The question has been carefully studied (see Sect. 7.3); there's no need to speculate when we have data.

I will point out when the data are meager, and often encourage your IRB to fill the evidentiary lacuna. This research would sometimes require little more than a willingness to examine the records your committee generates in its routine operations (see Sect. 9.1).

2.3   Scandal

We begin our discussion of ethics review with two notorious experiments at the heart of the IRB system's history.

In the 1950s, Chester Southam, a scientist at Sloan-Kettering in New York, began a series of experiments to understand our bodies' response to malignancies—how we fight off cancer or succumb to it. This promising research led Southam into moral failure when, in 1963, he injected live cancer cells into patients in the Jewish Chronic Disease Hospital in Brooklyn without their consent. His subjects suffered no significant physical harm but his violation of their dignity was shocking (Katz et al. 1972, p. 9–65).

The most infamous experiment of twentieth-century America was the Tuskegee syphilis study, which lasted from 1932 to 1972. During those 40 years, government doctors actively kept poor black sharecroppers with syphilis from obtaining treatment. The infection invaded their hearts and brains; some died. The scientists took careful notes.

2.4   Research Ethics

Even morally sound medical progress comes at a price. Polio vaccines could be developed only through trials that cost some children their lives. This research was not immoral, for the scientists used the safest methods available. In contrast, the effectiveness of new antibiotics was sometimes proven by withholding them from patients in need (Beecher 1966).

Research ethics, which examines the moral dimensions of research, blossomed in this time of promise and peril. Hans Jonas, a philosopher, Paul Ramsey, a theologian, and Henry K. Beecher, a doctor, were among the first in the field (Beecher 1966; Jonas 1969; Ramsey 1970). Beecher, the Henry Isaiah Dorr Professor of Anaesthesia Research at Harvard, exposed dozens of unethical investigations in his classic article (Beecher 1966); we will refer to it regularly.

We will also draw on the Belmont Report (National Commission 1978). One of the most respected documents in research ethics, the Report instructs your IRB to honor the moral principles of beneficence (concern for the welfare of others), respect for persons (concern for the rights of others), and justice.

Many aspects of research are ethically salient. Your IRB acts morally when it protects research subjects; scientists act morally when they discover new treatments for disease.

2.4.1   Two Ethical Principles

This manual rests on two ethical principles. As responsible people, we have (at least) two obligations:
• Do no harm to others, and
• Help others.

These obligations, which bind individuals and groups alike, are part of our social covenant. Your responsibility as a member of the IRB is shared by the other members, and your committee as a whole should act ethically. Similarly, your moral obligations extend to both individuals and groups.

2.4.2 Two Ethical Goals

The two principles translate directly into your IRB's two ethical goals: to protect subjects and to enable research that will benefit society.

Research ethics has traditionally focused on protecting human subjects from injury ("do no harm"), but that is only one piece of the picture. The other ethical centerpiece is the role of scholarly and scientific investigation in improving our health and our society ("help others"). It is, for instance, highly ethical to conduct research that reduces the burden of cancer, lessens the disparities in health between rich and poor, or exposes racial discrimination.

2.4.3 Goals into Practice

Much of the unethical research of the 1950s and 1960s was federally supported and a serious embarrassment for the funding agencies. James Shannon, director of the NIH, and his colleagues were determined to take action, but they faced a practical problem: what rules—what system—would block abusive studies without hindering ethically sound research? For an answer, they turned to a model close at hand.

NIH has its own hospital, the Clinical Center. In 1953, Center leaders formed the Clinical Research Committee to review potentially hazardous research (Frankel 1972, p. 10–12; Stark 2012, p. 75–77). This proto-IRB reduced but did not eliminate subject risk, allowing research that presented some risk so long as subjects were informed and gave their consent (Stark 2012).

The twin goals of the IRB system—safeguarding subject safety and enabling research intended to benefit the public—are a matter of historical record. In 1965, Shannon discussed the governance of science with a Public Health Service (PHS) advisory board. The PHS, Shannon said, planned to keep experiments on a sound ethical basis by means of "terms and conditions" that included the IRB system, which was only months from its launch. The PHS, he continued, had "a dual responsibility. One is a minor one of keeping the Government out of trouble … but really the major one is through these programs to try to encourage the development of terms and conditions that will encourage the flourishing of sound clinical investigation rather than discouraging it" (quoted in Frankel 1972, p. 31).

My belief that balanced review is essential rests not only on the historical record, but on societal expectations. The public, which was appalled at the research scandals of the postwar period, also relies on scientists to lessen the common burdens of our humanity.

In 1966, the PHS, under Shannon's leadership, directed institutions receiving agency funds to establish committees along the NIH model, thus creating the IRB system. Early IRBs were keenly interested in permitting research to proceed once they were confident that subject safety had been adequately safeguarded; they thus conducted balanced review.

2.4.4   Today's Loss of Balance

This balance has largely been lost (Brendel and Miller 2008); some authors even encourage IRBs to believe that their only concern should be subject safety. One manual asserts, "The regulatory mandate is clear: human subject protection, first, foremost, and last" (Shamoo and Khin-Maung-Gyi 2002, p. 58).

This statement would have been seen as bizarre at the system's birth; in 1966, nobody talked about subject protection as the IRB's sole concern. But by 1977, an observer remarked, "Peculiar to this time is the need to restate a proposition that, a decade ago, would have been regarded as self-evident, namely, that fostering excellence in medical research is in the public interest" (Eisenberg 1977).

Other ethicists have noted the contemporary tendency to focus exclusively on subjects. In 2007, a federal agency ruled that an experiment that found a new way to reduce hospital infections had violated the rights of its subjects. Ruth Faden, director of the Institute of Bioethics at Johns Hopkins, objected to this one-sided oversight: few people, she said, "have come forward to express concerns and oversight for the thirty thousand or so people who will die unnecessarily each year in the United States from this type of infection" (Faden et al. 2013). Her recognition of the value of research echoes the words of Hans Jonas, a philosopher who in 1969 praised science's struggle to combat disease and promote health and life. This "expansive goal," he said, has "the nobility of the free, forward thrust" (Jonas 1969, p. 230). Subjects themselves believe, sometimes passionately, that biomedical research saves lives, and they may be eager to participate even when it involves risk.

None of this is to say that social welfare should override individual rights. Jonas himself exhorted us never to permit subjects to be abused for the good of society (Jonas 1969). But when the question is not of abuse, but of risks that some subjects would willingly accept, the overprotection of subjects is an error. Educator and ethicist Rosamond Rhodes asks us not to try to protect subjects "from *any* risks, regardless of how unlikely, fleeting, or trivial the anticipated harm. When the physical and other risks involved are negligible and unlikely, and the study promises to provide a societal benefit, a reasonable assessment should conclude that the balance tips toward promoting scientific advance" (Rhodes 2014, emphasis in original).

2.4.5 It's Always About People

The balance your IRB should seek can be expressed in two ways: as "subject welfare versus scientific advances" or as "subject welfare versus societal benefit." Rhodes includes both formulations because they are not identical. For your IRB, science matters, not in its own right, but because it helps people. Scientific advances are a means to the end of societal benefit.

Successful biomedical scientists enjoy funding, promotion, and prestige, but these are only proxies for the value they create. Their work attains moral power because their discoveries save lives and reduce suffering. Similarly, research in the social sciences matters because society benefits when scholars expose plagues like racial discrimination. When I discuss the IRB's duty to "permit research to be conducted," that is a contraction for "permit research that will increase the well-being of society."

The word "society" is itself a contraction. Your IRB's duty is to the individuals who form society—to all of us as we struggle with illness, care for others, and confront injustice. Political philosopher Alan Wertheimer astutely observes, "It is often said that medical research exhibits a tension between science or progress or a 'greater social good' and the interests or rights of the individual. Although that way of putting things is not wrong, it is also misleading. After all, 'society,' and 'science,' and 'progress' do not describe metaphysical entities that are not reducible to the interests of individuals. Rather, they are different ways of describing the interests of discrete, albeit statistical, individuals." This does not resolve the ethical choices your IRB must make. "There may sometimes be a tension between the interests of individuals who serve as research subjects and the interests of individuals who stand to gain from such research. But it's individuals versus individuals all the way down" (Wertheimer 2011, p. 5).

Your IRB will have constant contact with scientists and scholars. They deserve every opportunity to achieve their professional goals. But their primary claim on your ethical judgment is derivative of the need of the people, unknown and perhaps unborn, who will benefit.

Dennis Mazur, who is a professor of medicine, senior scholar in ethics, and long-time IRB chair, cautions your IRB against becoming "a force for the promotion of research" (Mazur 2007, p. 222). Mazur is right on two counts. While research is important, subject protection must never be forgotten. Further, your IRB never actively promotes research; you merely make it possible for others to conduct it, by protecting subjects from harm, facilitating informed subject choice, and providing scientists with an objective third party to guard them from error.

2.5   Ethical Goals and Regulatory Means

Your IRB's decisions should be respected because they are ethically persuasive; they must be obeyed because you hold federal power. You pursue ethical goals through regulatory means.

2.5.1   Principles of Regulation

Regulation, like ethics, has its own principles. Responsible regulators honor these virtues:
- Respectfulness
- Transparency, by operating on the basis of rules that are known to all
- Efficiency, by seeking maximal benefit at least cost to all parties
- Clarity, by using language in ways that make communication easy

- Accountability, by justifying their decisions and reconsidering them when questioned
- Judiciousness, able to distinguish significant from trivial
- Rationality, striving to improve the public interest in ways that are based on evidence
- Restraint, acting only within the scope of their authority

These principles are discussed in Sect. 3.1. Your IRB should follow both ethical and regulatory best practices.

2.5.2 *Organization and Legal Framework*

Your IRB is part of a multitiered system of oversight (Halpern 2008). You look over the scientist's shoulder, and government officials look over yours.

During the 1970s and 1980s, federal funding agencies realized that they had no method in place to protect subjects. Multiple agencies implemented rules for ethics review, no two alike; IRBs struggled to keep track of which agency required what. This regulatory jumble was unsnarled in 1991, when the Department of Health and Human Services (HHS) and 14 other federal departments and agencies agreed that all would follow a single set of regulations; this is known as the Common Rule (45 CFR 46 Subpart A). The FDA simultaneously modified its regulations to be nearly identical to the Common Rule (21 CFR 50 and 56).

The OHRP, which is within the NIH, and the FDA have primary responsibility for oversight of IRB operations. Your committee's relationship with these two agencies is central to your effective functioning (see Chap. 8 for more on this topic). Your IRB may also be guided by state or local regulations, which are outside the scope of this manual.

2.6 Your IRB Service

You should be proud of your work on the IRB, but pride should not be your only reward. You should serve on equitable terms, fairly compensated and adequately protected.

2.6.1   Compensation

In some institutions, IRB service is undemanding, but many IRBs have long meetings (2 or 3 h is not uncommon) with substantial additional time spent in preparation. Joining the IRB is a significant commitment.

If you are not yet a member, you need to decide if the terms you are offered make sense. If you are a junior faculty member, your department may require committee service as a condition for tenure, but excessive time spent outside your core responsibilities will jeopardize your future. Many IRBs require far more work than any other institutional committee.

Some institutions pay IRB members for their service, either in cash or by releasing them from other obligations. Others do not, on the ground that everyone has an obligation to participate in the institution's governance; this approach may be revisited if new members prove hard to recruit.

If your department chair indicates that he or she will be grateful if you agree to serve, ask if that gratitude will be manifested in some concrete fashion. Pediatrician and ethicist Daniel Nelson advises that the institution "should send a clear signal that IRB membership is a necessary and important activity and recognize such service when considering promotions, tenure, and clinical work schedules" (Nelson 2011, p. 108). One particularly welcome signal is for the institution to pay your department for time spent on IRB duties, so that the department can compensate you.

If you are invited to serve on the IRB and are unsure what to do, contact current committee members and ask what their service is like. Be a good citizen but not a martyr.

If you are the non-affiliated, non-scientist, or community member, some institutions won't pay you, some will, and some will only if you ask. Some community members enjoy their service and don't mind being unpaid; others will not work without compensation. It's your choice.

2.6.2   Protection from Lawsuits

It is unusual for IRB members to be sued for their work on the committee, but it does happen (Halikas v. Minnesota 1996; Icenogle 2003; Berrett 2011; Looney v. Moore 2013). Your institution should promise to furnish you with legal defense and pay any financial penalty assessed against you (Nelson 2011). I will wager that the members of the Board of Trustees have this protection as they undertake their official duties. Have they extended it to you?

2.6.3 The Community Member

Every IRB must have at least one member who is not affiliated with the institution and at least one member who is not a scientist (21 CFR 56.108(c-d), 45 CFR 46.107(c-d)). Many IRBs use a single person, an unaffiliated nonscientist, to fulfill both roles. A member who serves in either or both roles is often called the community member, although the regulations do not use that term.

Commentators do not agree on what the role of the community member should be (Klitzman 2012a). In 1969, when the IRB system was rapidly evolving, legal scholar Guido Calabresi speculated that the doctors on review boards would be reluctant to expose subjects to significant risks. The nonscientists, Calabresi guessed, "would tend, on the whole, to approve some experiments that would not now be passed. This is especially true where the potential gains from an experiment are great, but the risks involved are also great." He predicted that lay people would be less inclined than doctors to fear lawsuits or to feel there was a special obligation to the subject, and "more likely to give greater weight to society's long-run interest" (Calabresi 1969, p. 400). Thirty years later, the National Bioethics Advisory Commission took the opposite position, seeing the community member as representing potential research participants, not society at large (National Bioethics Advisory Commission 2001, p. xvi).

In the absence of consensus, you as a community member can serve in any way that makes sense to you and your IRB chair. Your contributions, like those of every other member, will be dictated by your abilities. If you are a high school art teacher and every other member of the committee is a medical specialist, you are unlikely to understand the protocols in the same depth as they. You don't have to, and that is not why you are here. You bring an outsider's perspective that the board needs.

Robert Levine, the Yale scholar who is one of the IRB system's intellectual architects, expresses the proper role of the community member beautifully. "The layperson-members should be assured that each and every IRB member is a part of the laity with regard to the specialties of some or all others. They should work together in a climate of trust that each will contribute according to his or her abilities to the overall function of the IRB" (Levine 2006b, p. 61–62).

2.7   The Triumph of Ethics Review

From the start, the IRB system dramatically reduced unethical experiments, including those that enlisted subjects without their consent (Curran 1969). Jerry Menikoff, before he became head of OHRP, wrote, "By any standard, it must be recognized there has been a massive change with regard to informed consent, and all for the better." The problems of unethical research in the 1960s, "people being enrolled in studies without their even knowing they were in a study ... seem to be from a very different world" (Menikoff and Richards 2006, p. 85).

The best-documented example of a successful early IRB was at Case Western, where the dean of the medical school led the committee and the members were all department chairs. This committee conducted careful review without unduly encumbering research (Cowan 1974). Research subjects no longer had to trust the integrity of the investigator, because someone else was looking after the subject's welfare. This is the triumph of ethics review. It is an important contribution to society, and I hope it is one of the reasons you are willing to serve on the IRB.

Chapter 3
IRB Process

We move now from lofty theory to pedestrian practice. This chapter focuses on the process your committee uses; later chapters address the science and scholarship you review. I use the phrase "science and scholarship" as shorthand for the major branches of knowledge under review: biomedical science, largely conducted in hospitals and medical schools, and the social sciences as found in colleges and universities.

3.1 Principles

When your IRB embodies the virtues of responsible regulation (see Sect. 2.5), you demonstrate that your operations are fair. These principles also facilitate wise decisions.

3.1.1 Respectfulness

Your IRB should respect the investigators you assist. This is no mere courtesy; it is a duty for any person vested with federal power.

Psychiatrist and ethicist Robert Klitzman interviewed IRB chairs from across the United States; some acknowledged that they may seem "harsh and potentially insensitive" to investigators. One said, "We have a little bit of a reputation of grilling the investigators when they come in, and I think they're a little bit nervous when they walk in.

© Springer International Publishing Switzerland 2016
S.N. Whitney, *Balanced Ethics Review*,
DOI 10.1007/978-3-319-20705-6_3

But I don't think that's necessarily bad, because I don't think every-body should feel like it's a cake walk—that everything's going to get passed" (Klitzman 2011b).

This is not how one member of a university or medical school should treat another. You and the scientists and scholars whose work you review are colleagues.

The respect should be mutual. I know of investigators who treat the IRB, and everything else in their path, with contempt, asserting that their board is incapable of understanding their protocols or pro-viding constructive suggestions. This is irresponsible.

Scientists with concerns about the IRB should speak with the chair. Scientists who do not realize that the IRB's flexibility is limited by federal (and sometimes state) regulations should become better informed. Scientists who feel the regulations themselves are defective should campaign for their reform. Scientists with persistent questions about the IRB should not be surprised if they are invited to join.

3.1.2 Transparency

Your IRB is transparent when its operations are visible to the public. Every IRB should have a website on which it posts its:
* Members
* Meeting times and places
* Standard operating procedures
* Minutes
* Sample consent forms and approved protocols

Your IRB's meetings should be open (Klitzman 2011b). Joan Sieber and Martin Tolich (Sieber and Tolich 2013, p. 209), both expe-rienced IRB chairs, believe that "the researcher should have the right to appear before the IRB, and the IRB should account in person for its decisions."

There is a time for secrecy even in the deliberation of public bod-ies; IRBs are justified in protecting proprietary information and the details of legal disputes. But nobody has provided a rationale for extending secrecy beyond limited areas like these.

3.1.3 Efficiency

A scholar I know once told his IRB that the revisions it required would drain his budget. "Cost is not our concern," a member replied.

This attitude is encouraged by the literature. One article argues that stringent regulation "should be encouraged and supported even if it will increase administrative burden and delay the research. Efficiency itself is not a moral imperative or an ethical value, and we believe that human subjects protections should never be compromised by a desire for increased efficiency" (Davis and Hurley 2014, p. 17–18).

Efficiency is not an ethical value but it can serve ethical ends. As Leon Eisenberg notes, the "imposition of impediments to significant therapeutic research is itself unethical because an important benefit is being denied to the community" (Eisenberg 1977). If your IRB bears cost in mind, it will do wonders for your reputation.

3.1.4 Clarity

Research ethics has its own conventions and ways of using language. These are generally helpful, but one, the concept of coercion, has led to confusion.

Some of the literature mistakenly considers encouragement or persuasion to be equivalent to coercion. IRBs can be tripped up on this point; one committee determined that it was coercive for a brochure to use the word "hope" in a discussion of what subjects hope for when they enroll in a study (Getz 2011). You should shun this incorrect usage, for mere optimism has nothing to do with coercion. The distinguished philosopher Tom Beauchamp explains that "coercion occurs if and only if one person intentionally uses a credible and severe threat of harm or force to control another" (Beauchamp 2010, p. 69). Follow Beauchamp's lead.

3.1.5   Accountability

Your IRB should provide for appeals (Sieber and Tolich 2013, p. 210). You can use any method that complies with the regulations (appeals cannot be to a higher institutional official (45 CFR 46.112)) and suits your circumstances.

The first step might be a request for reconsideration by the original board. A robust process would also provide for recourse to a suitably-constituted appellate IRB, either in the host institution or in another, so that a fresh opinion may be formed (Lantos 2007b).

3.1.6   Judiciousness

Every protocol has points of ethical interest; each touches, in one way or another, on our commitment to protecting subjects and our hopes for better lives. But not every protocol raises ethical issues that require IRB intervention. If most of the protocols your IRB reviews are relatively safe, they should require minimal intervention. Discipline yourself to focus on protocols that pose substantive ethical issues.

In the absence of significant problems, it is tempting to require minor changes to demonstrate your diligence (Levine 2006a; Baron 2015). Australian anthropologist Maureen Fitzgerald, who studied ethics review in five countries, was struck that "there seems to be some need among committee members to make some comment or request some action"; otherwise "there is a sense that they are not fulfilling their responsibilities as a committee" (Fitzgerald et al. 2006). Rubin observed that IRBs "'must' find something wrong with each and every application, so as to generate a paper trail proving the thoroughness of their review." As a result, "enormous effort is now expended on routine and mundane protocols" (Rubin 2001).

Your committee should avoid busywork, not serve as its headwaters.

3.1.7 Rationality

Ethics review is not a purely rational affair; judgment, experience, and intuition all play a role. But your memory and intuition should yield to published evidence when it is available. This manual draws on evidence from the ethics literature whenever possible; you should do likewise.

3.1.8 Restraint

Your IRB should refrain from exceeding the bounds of its authority, a phenomenon that is aptly called mission creep. Mission creep is a manifestation of the curse of power—an important and common problem that merits separate discussion.

3.2 The Curse of Power

Your IRB has dominion over dozens or hundreds of scientists and scholars; you approve or reject hundreds or thousands of requests annually. Your IRB is, in a word, powerful.

You were given this power for an important purpose: to protect the rights and welfare of subjects. But the regulations do not say that you must restrict your attention to this goal; and because your committee has plenary power over research with humans, well-meaning people will attempt to hijack you into pursuing their goals.

Their perspective is understandable. Almost any failure in research can be cast in ethical terms. People who see a shortcoming in science or scholarship, and know of your power, will naturally call on you to remedy the problem.

Their concern may be valid, but unless the problem involves protecting the rights and welfare of subjects, it is outside your jurisdiction. British scientist Ian Chalmers, for instance, has called on IRBs to "use their powers to reduce unnecessary research—which, by definition, cannot be ethical." He is particularly troubled by research that "is proposed for perverse reasons, reflecting the interests of industry and academia more than those of patients" (Chalmers 2007). No doubt some research is frivolous, but I advise you against trying to divine whether commercial or academic research will ultimately benefit patients; the problem is not yours to solve. Your mission is to make sure it does not compromise the interests of subjects.

3.2.1   Scope of IRB Authority

The curse of power is at its most seductive when people urge you to expand the scope of your protection. Resist their blandishments.

Your IRB should protect only subjects.

Nobody else.

Period.

Do Not Protect Third Parties. In some interview and social science research, subjects may mention friends, family members, and other people. This could lead to embarrassment or worse (Hadjistavropoulos and Smythe 2001), but your IRB was created to protect subjects, not anyone they happen to mention (see Sects. 6.5 and 6.6).

Do Not Protect Scientists. Some authors urge you to protect scientists (Smith 1999, p. 94–96; Sieber and Tolich 2013, p. 190–191) but without justifying your taking on this additional responsibility.

Ruth Armstrong (Armstrong et al. 2014) was a graduate student in criminology who wanted to study how convicts adapt to their new lives after they are released from prison. The IRB that reviewed her research knew almost nothing about these parolees or Armstrong herself. Nonetheless, it felt that she should meet them somewhere safe, a request that brings to mind a coffee shop in a nice neighborhood. The committee seemed unaware that if she requested such a meeting place it would signal mistrust and imperil her research.

The IRB has the power but not the authority to protect the scholar. She, her advisor, and her department are responsible for her safety.

Do Not Protect Research Assistants. Sieber and Tolich urge IRBs to protect "invisible, powerless, and vulnerable research assistants" from threats ranging from physical assault to the emotional trauma of transcribing distressing interviews. They recommend that when someone is hired as a contract researcher, the IRB ask if they should be treated "as a participant in the research" and given their own consent form. The IRB can then ensure that the job description is detailed and spells out all "likely emotional and physical harms." The IRB should review the terms of employment: Is the pay fair? Is counseling support available? If so, is it free and confidential? Is the safety plan adequate? (Sieber and Tolich 2013, p. 178).

The mistake here is imagining that the research assistant should be treated like a participant in the research. This opens the door to the IRB scrutinizing the assistant's wages, working conditions, and mental health.

The assistant is not a research participant, and none of this is any of the IRB's business. The investigator who hires the assistant, and the university's human resources department, are responsible for employee safety and terms of employment. The regulations do not even remotely contemplate the IRB second guessing this process.

Do Not Protect Communities. Philosopher Charles Weijer and ethicist Ezekiel Emanuel urge IRBs to protect communities from the harmful impact of biomedical research. They worry, for example, that research into particular genetic mutations may expose communities such as the Ashkenazi Jews to discrimination (Weijer and Emanuel 2000). Their concern is understandable, and the scientists should take the welfare of the communities they study to heart. The IRB, however, has no duty to protect communities from the results of research.

Do Not Protect Companies. As part of her pathbreaking research in IRB functioning, sociologist Laura Stark interviewed 18 IRB chairs about a study that might show that some firms were discriminating against racial minorities (see Sect. 6.7 for the details). Some chairs were uneasy about the research, and one wanted to protect employers from being exposed as discriminatory (Stark 2012, p. 44). It is unethical to shield people who act immorally (and illegally) from exposure; but companies are not even people, and thus are beyond the IRB's remit.

3.2.2 Litigation Prevention

Your IRB should not attempt to identify and parry legal threats in the protocols you review. Nothing in the letter or spirit of the regulations suggests that IRBs are responsible for protecting their universities from litigation, and institutions have better ways to defend themselves.

The IRBs that Stark studied nonetheless required protocol changes "to safeguard the investigator, the board itself, or the university from lawsuits or legal reprimand" (Stark 2006, p. 184). The chair mentioned above brought up this concern with regard to research intended to see if companies discriminate on the basis of race, arguing "that there were serious legal risks to the employers being studied if the investigator breached confidentiality and it became known publicly that certain employers were discriminating against job candidates." She commented, "I can imagine that if you're someone accused of discrimination, you're going to pursue this and sue the researcher" (227).

Let's unpack this. A company that routinely rejected minority job seekers could file a suit against the investigator, presumably for libel, but few firms would welcome the negative publicity that would follow. A truthful statement is not libelous, so the employer would likely lose in court. Finally, it is against federal law to discriminate on the basis of race.

Most IRBs have neither the training nor the authority to guard against legal threats. If you are concerned that research could lead to litigation you should refer the matter to the appropriate institutional official.

One final hazard merits mention. At least two IRBs have been sued by researchers who felt their research was being improperly encumbered (Halikas v. Minnesota 1996; Berrett 2011). Your best protection is to conduct fair and balanced review.

3.2.3   Beyond the Regulations

The curse of power is made possible by the indeterminacy of the regulations, which say what your IRB must do but set no limits on what you may do. In addition to expanding the scope of your activities, as discussed above, you are free to impose requirements on investigators beyond those specified by the regulations. Should you?

Ethics review consultants Amy Davis and Elisa Hurley argue that "IRBs should never be required to report or justify additional measures they adopt to augment protection of human subjects. Federal regulations are considered *minimum* standards for protection, and in our view, to exceed those standards should be encouraged and supported" (Davis and Hurley 2014, p. 17–18, emphasis in original). This belief, often accompanied by the phrase that regulations are "the floor, not the ceiling," is regularly presented as self-evidently sound policy (Levine 1986, p. 342; Russell-Einhorn and Ellis 1998; Cohen 2010).

These comments assume that subject protection matters and the common good does not; but your IRB should consider the welfare of both subjects and society. If you can find a way to enhance the protection of subjects without damaging research, you should do so, but you must always bear cost in mind. When a significant cost yields a trivial benefit, exceeding the regulatory requirements is an ethical error.

Chapter 4
Evaluating Biomedical Research

Your IRB conducts ethical review of biomedical investigations. To evaluate a study you must have a reasonable understanding of the science, since the ethics of a protocol flow from its particularities; those details will lead you to approve, modify, or reject it.

4.1 The Objective IRB

Your committee has scientists, but it is unlikely to understand any given study as well as the investigators who wrote it. This is not a defect; it is an inherent feature of IRB review, and your distance is an asset as you evaluate a protocol's ethics. You are not reviewing protocols because you are more ethical than the researchers, but because you are more objective. Investigators, however ethical and well-intentioned, have interests that may distort their judgment (Ramsey 1970; Emanuel et al. 2000).

4.1.1 Ramsey and the Scientist's Bias

Early ethicists observed scientists' lack of detachment from the moral content of their work. Paul Ramsey, who was Professor of Religion at Princeton, was particularly struck by the reluctance of scientists to allow subject consent to slow their investigations. "The researcher knows that his judgment will generally be biased by the fact that he

© Springer International Publishing Switzerland 2016
S.N. Whitney, *Balanced Ethics Review*,
DOI 10.1007/978-3-319-20705-6_4

strongly desires one of the consequences (the rapid completion of his research for the good of mankind) which he could hope to attain by breaking or avoiding the requirement of an informed consent. ... If every doer loves his deed more than it ought to be loved, so every researcher his research—and, of course, its promise of future benefits for mankind" (Ramsey 1970, p. 10). As befits a theologian, Ramsey describes the moral pitfalls of science in the abstract; but his words nail the immorality of the cancer cell injections, in which Southam surely loved his experiment too much (see Sect. 2.2).

Ramsey's memorable antidote to this bias is a kind of self-coaching. "The investigator should strive, as Aristotle suggested, to hit the mean of moral virtue or excellence by 'leaning against' the excess or the defect to which he knows himself, individually or professionally, and mankind generally in a scientific age, to be especially inclined" (10).

No doubt some scientists follow this practice; the IRB system is premised on the assumption that some do not. Your committee ensures that subjects are protected even when the scientist would like to take a shortcut, and you do this without being an expert.

4.1.2   Your Reasonable Understanding

Some authors believe that the IRB must be able to understand each protocol in sufficient depth to make an independent and accurate assessment of every aspect. One manual urges your committee to check the qualifications of the scientists, to assess "scientific issues such as significance of preliminary data, feasibility of specific aims, and data analysis plans," and to "fully consider the procedures involved in research" (Khan and Kornetsky 2005, p. 120, 122).

Don't take this seriously. Your IRB is unlikely to achieve an in-depth comprehension of the disease being studied, its treatment, the methods used to evaluate a new remedy, and the statistics that will prove or disprove its efficacy. You don't have to. Neither ethics nor the regulations require you to become an expert in every biomedical niche; you need only the reasonable understanding that will allow you to protect subjects.

4.2 Literature Reviews

Scientists need to be in command of their fields. Some IRBs therefore require the investigator to submit a review of the literature with each application. This requirement goes beyond what the regulations demand—an example of the curse of power (see Sect. 3.2.3)—and neither the FDA nor OHRP has imposed a review of the literature as a new obligation. There is also no evidence that this practice improves subject protection.

4.2.1 Death at Johns Hopkins

A tragic story drives IRB requests for literature reviews. In 2001, a scientist at Johns Hopkins used hexamethonium, a chemical that usually induces a mild asthmatic reaction, to study the body's bronchial defenses. Ellen Roche, a lab technician at the Asthma Center, volunteered to participate; the chemical caused a fatal reaction.

Her response should not have been a surprise. Hexamethonium was once used as a prescription medication, but the FDA withdrew its approval after serious reactions were documented in the literature. The Johns Hopkins investigator and IRB were unaware of this history. A thorough literature search, by either the investigator or the IRB, might have uncovered this evidence and saved Roche's life.

4.2.2 Reviews by Investigators

After Roche's death, many IRBs began requiring scientists to submit literature reviews with their applications. Investigators certainly need to have a comprehensive understanding of any medication or procedure that they will use, but there is no published evidence that a mandatory literature search adds to the investigator's fund of knowledge or assists the IRB in its deliberations.

If there is an IRB that routinely studies the literature reviews produced by investigators to assist its deliberations, it should share its insights in print. If there are scientists who find IRB-required literature reviews to be helpful, their experiences should be documented. If these reviews are filed and forgotten, the practice should be abandoned.

4.2.3   Reviews by IRBs

Dennis Mazur urges the IRB itself to conduct literature reviews as standard practice. "Each IRB member must learn how to search the peer-reviewed medical literature"; such searches "must become a routine part of an IRB member's fulfillment of the role" (Mazur 2007, p. 114, 224). Conducting the search is only the beginning. "The results of a basic search should be reviewed with local experts, for instance, to extend the list of known risks. Clinical experts, by attending medical society meetings that report and discuss recent research, may have learned of risks before they appear in the medical literature" (115).

No IRB could routinely meet this standard, and I have found no evidence that this could produce benefits to justify the heroic investment of time it would require. If Mazur's IRB is conducting regular literature reviews, it should publish its methods and results so that we can all learn from it.

You should invest enough time to attain a working understanding of the research you review, and there is no reason to restrict yourself to the information provided in the protocol; you can, for instance, contact the investigator or query outside experts. On a case-by-case basis, you may also do your own review of the literature, but you should feel no obligation to do so.

4.3   Ethics and Science

Your IRB can approve a protocol, approve it with modifications, or reject it. You are cognizant of the science but focus on the ethics.

4.3.1 Scientific Modifications

Some IRBs are charged by the institution with critiquing the methodology of the protocols they review. These committees play an active role in training young scientists, improving the quality of investigations, and conserving institutional resources. If your IRB is responsible for scientific oversight, then modifying the protocols you review is part of your expanded mission. You may point out flaws in the protocol, or you may take a more active role by suggesting—or insisting on—specific remedies.

Some experts believe that even IRBs that do not serve as scientific review boards have a duty to ensure that the quality of the science is optimized (Amdur 2011), and many IRBs require changes of many of the protocols they review (Fitzgerald et al. 2006; Stark 2012). They assume that if they can do anything to improve the protocol, they should; but this plausible assumption is not grounded in evidence. There has been no systematic review of IRB modifications of scientific proposals; we are therefore left with anecdotes, and they are hardly encouraging. Too often, well-intentioned modifications delay and damage research (Gunsalus et al. 2007). There is no harm in making suggestions. But if you expect your suggestions to be followed, that may reflect power more than wisdom.

If your IRB, which is not charged with conducting scientific review, routinely modifies research, you should either stop or study your own process. This could be done as follows:

1. Identify the three to five kinds of protocols your committee deals with most frequently.
2. Establish a panel of experts in each of those areas.
3. Pull a sample of protocols of each type as submitted and as approved after your modifications.
4. Circulate both versions to the experts, without indicating which were before review and which after.
5. Ask the experts which version is scientifically better, and why.

4.3.2 The Value of Research

Your IRB may reject a proposal for a variety of reasons, including your belief that the investigation is without value. NIH bioethicists

Ezekiel Emanuel, David Wendler, and Christine Grady encourage you to use this power, on the grounds that subjects should never be exposed to risk for research that is not "socially or scientifically" valuable. This would include "clinical research with nongeneraliz-able results, a trifling hypothesis, or substantial or total overlap with proven results. In addition, research with results unlikely to be dis-seminated or in which the intervention could never be practically implemented even if effective is not valuable" (Emanuel et al. 2000). Their recommendation echoes Ian Chalmers's advice that you reject research that may not benefit patients (see Sect. 3.2).

I agree that it is unethical to expose subjects to risk as part of an experiment that cannot produce useful results. But if your IRB is not an expert, you may find it challenging to determine whether results can be generalized or a hypothesis is important. It is also unclear that you should, in the rapidly changing world of medicine, reject research that might overlap with proven results. Scientists can profit-ably probe the "safety, effectiveness, efficiency, accessibility and quality" of even proven interventions (World Medical Association.). An IRB that regularly rejects research because it is worthless would perform a great service by publishing a series of its decisions.

This discussion assumes the research imposes significant risk. It is ethical for subjects to participate in research whose results may never be published but that is harmless or offers a possibility of individual benefit, like a program that offers schoolchildren assistance with diet and exercise.

4.3.3 Risk

Fifty years ago, it was all too common for research to pose unaccept-able hazards (Beecher 1966), so early IRBs probably had ample opportunities to reduce the risk to subjects. Donald Chalkley, chief of the NIH's Institutional Relations Section (forerunner to today's OHRP), reported in 1968 on federal data about proposals for NIH funding that presented "medical, psychological, or sociological" haz-ards. Chalkley said that in 1966, 7.4 % of proposals were "problem projects" (quoted in Curran 1969). An IRB of that era would have had its hands full.

Scientists got the message. Within 2 years, Chalkley reported, there had been a "dramatic" decline to 1.7 % (quoted in Curran 1969). Unfortunately, federal authorities stopped collecting this data; perhaps there was no longer a perceived need.

Your IRB was created to identify problem projects. In 1966, if Chalkley's numbers are accurate, one proposal in 14 would have been problematic. By 1968 the proportion had dropped to 1 in 60. By 1981, Robert Levine could write, "Much of the literature on the ethics of research involving human subjects reflects the widely held and, until recently, unexamined assumption that playing the role of research subject is a highly perilous business." But, he added, the data "indicate that, in general, it is not particularly hazardous to be a research subject" (Levine 1981, p. 25).

Levine's comment, and contemporary data, reflect a transformation in how scientists design research. There will always be hazardous protocols, but they are far less common than when the system was founded.

4.4 Weighing Risks, Benefits, and Knowledge

The regulations require your IRB, before it approves a protocol, to determine that "risks to subjects are reasonable in relation to anticipated benefits, if any, to subjects, and the importance of the knowledge that may reasonably be expected to result" (45 CFR 46.111(a) (2)). This may be your most difficult task.

One problem is that you often lack trustworthy estimates of risk and benefit (more on this later); another is the variability in how subjects themselves see risk and benefit. As Dennis Mazur points out, "The IRB must assess how reasonable the risks are in a study according to a range of personal preferences that participants might have regarding the risks. ... A person's past and current experiences related to his or her medical conditions, disease processes, past and current care, and past and recent research experiences may give a potential participant a dramatically different view of the severity of risk from that of an expert, the principal investigator, or IRB member" (Mazur 2007, p. 72, 69). In fact, as bioethicist Michelle Meyer shows, a single study may be seen as offering net benefit by one subject and net harm by another (Meyer 2014).

Altruism can play a decisive role. Some prospective subjects, learning that a study requires a lumbar puncture (spinal tap), might refuse because they have had a miserable experience with that procedure. Others might enroll because their experience was less miserable, they consider the research important, and they realize that a study involving a lumbar puncture might struggle to recruit enough people.

Some of the problem of variability is naturally resolved by the consent process. If your IRB approves a protocol with a reasonable mixture of risks and benefits, some subjects will consent, others will decline. But how risky a project can you approve? In making this judgment, you implicitly balance two of the Belmont Report principles, beneficence and respect for persons. Beneficence (concern for another's welfare) directs you to protect prospective subjects from risks that you feel are excessive; respect for persons encourages you to allow subjects to choose for themselves, based on the risks as they see them. We will review the arguments for each of these approaches in turn.

4.4.1 Why You Should Protect Subjects

Protecting subjects is in your IRB's blood; Title II of the law that animates the system is called "Protection of Human Subjects" (National Research Service Award Act of 1974). This is not the curse of power; it is why you have power.

When we let subjects choose, we rely on them to make sound decisions, presumably on the basis of the information provided as part of the consent process. But skeptical observers have long doubted that consent could protect subjects from harm. Beecher assumed that purported consent to risky research was invalid (Beecher 1966), and Franz Ingelfinger mocked informed consent as a myth. Ingelfinger, then editor of the *New England Journal of Medicine*, asked us to "assume that the experimental subject, whether a patient, a volunteer, or otherwise enlisted, is exposed to a completely honest array of factual detail." After he is so exposed, what does his consent mean? "With his written signature, the subject then caps the transaction, and whether he sees himself as a heroic martyr for the sake of mankind, or as a reluctant guinea pig dragooned for the benefit of science, or whether, perhaps, he is merely bewildered, he obviously has given his 'informed consent'" (Ingelfinger 1972).

Ruth Faden led the Advisory Committee on Human Radiation Experiments, which interviewed research participants in depth. Her interviewees considered the consent process to be unimportant, and decided whether to participate based on their attitudes toward the investigator and institution. Faden concluded that it is "naïve to think that informed consent can be relied upon as the major mechanism to protect the rights and interests of patient-subjects" (Advisory Committee 1996, p. 484–485).

If consent is not enough, IRBs must themselves weigh risks and benefits. As they do, they are conservative, which is not only prudent, it is the emphatic preference of the FDA and OHRP (see Chap. 8). Caution is also supported by the Belmont Report, for when you reject a hazardous protocol, you honor the Belmont principle of beneficence by promoting subject safety.

4.4.2 Why You Should Let Subjects Choose

But invoking beneficence does not settle the matter. A narrow view of beneficence focuses on subject safety; a broader view recognizes that subjects have their own views of their rights and welfare and that their attitudes toward money, altruism, and risk may differ from yours. Further, the Belmont Report principle of respect for persons encourages you to allow subjects more choice, lest you protect them more than they wish.

These considerations, which would have been irrelevant during the unethical research of the 1960s, grew in force as dangerous proposals diminished. At the same time that Levine commented that it is "not particularly hazardous to be a research subject," he wrote, "when considering particular proposals to involve autonomous adults as research subjects, if I must err, I am inclined to err on the side of autonomy. This is because I consider overprotection to be a form of disrespect for persons" (Levine 1981, p. 47).

What Levine calls overprotection is done by IRBs who, with good intentions, face the impossible task of determining whether unmeasured risks and uncertain benefits would be appropriate for unknown subjects. People tend to be more cautious about allowing others to take risks than they would be for themselves; a committee making a decision about the welfare of another person is likely to be particularly risk averse (Atanasov 2010). IRBs thus tend, writes Michelle Meyer, "through a broad understanding of research risk and a narrow understanding of research benefit, to make risk-benefit decisions that reflect the (imagined) preferences of the most vulnerable, risk-averse participants" (Meyer 2014, p. 322). Maureen Fitzgerald observed this in practice, writing of committee members imagining a "*what if* or *worst case narrative*" that can be made iteratively more dire until it "may significantly overestimate the kind, potential for, probability of, or seriousness of the risk" (Fitzgerald et al. 2006, emphasis in original).

By 2005, Rosamond Rhodes objected that our "well-meaning efforts" may be "misdirected and counter-productive in that many may do more harm than good in terms of safeguarding personal autonomy and supporting autonomous choices" (Rhodes 2005).

4.4.3 The Conundrum

We thus arrive at a central quandary of research ethics, with eminent experts urging us in opposite directions. Your IRB may seem doomed to commit either the sin of neglect (by allowing subjects to make too-risky choices) or of paternalism (by thwarting subject autonomy). You cannot refuse the choice; it is what you do.

4.5 Approval Based on Risk and Benefit

Recall the regulatory instructions: your IRB must ensure that "risks to subjects are reasonable in relation to anticipated benefits, if any, to subjects, and the importance of the knowledge that may reasonably be expected to result" (45 CFR 46 .111(a)(2)). It sounds so simple. True, the regulations provide no detailed instructions on how to weigh risks, benefits, and knowledge, but that is presumably what your committee has been brought together to do.

The problem is that you lack the information to make the judgment. Now and then you will have reliable data, but usually risks are approximate, benefits are speculative, and the importance of the knowledge to be gained may remain murky even after the study is published. As a result, there is no generally accepted way to determine when a protocol's risks and benefits justify your permitting subjects to enroll. There is, instead, a thicket of competing theories, none with substantial empirical support.

4.5.1 Established Theories

Emanuel, Wendler, and Grady, while conceding that the analysis cannot be quantitative, defend the concept of balancing risk and benefit even in the absence of a formula. This assessment "can appeal to explicit standards, informed by existing data on the potential types of harms and benefits, their likelihood of occurring, and their long-term consequences" (Emanuel et al. 2000). Charles Weijer (with Paul Miller) presents an alternative approach, proposing that IRBs undertake a "component analysis" of the risks of research, distinguishing procedures that have a therapeutic intent from those that do not (Weijer 2000; Weijer and Miller 2004). David Wendler and his NIH colleague Franklin Miller suggest a third approach, the "net risks test," that puts IRBs "in a position to protect participants without blocking appropriate research studies" (Wendler and Miller 2007).

These are all reasonable suggestions, but there is little evidence that IRBs follow them. Laura Stark (Stark 2006, 2012) observed three IRBs over a prolonged period; in none of the many discussions she describes does the committee list the likelihood and impact of the risks and benefits to subjects, factor in the likely benefit to society, and balance them to reach a reasoned decision. I know of no IRB that has systematically followed any of these approaches in its everyday operations and published a series of cases showing how the method succeeded or failed. We are rich in theory but paupers in evidence.

In the absence of a workable method, IRBs do the best they can. Robert Klitzman learned that committee members rely on their "gut feelings" and "intuition," occasionally using "the sniff test" to determine if research should be approved (Klitzman 2011a, b). This is a wretched way to make important decisions, but in the absence of clear guidance, it is not the IRB's fault. As you strive to anticipate the hopes and fears of people you will never meet, you are likely to rely, uncomfortably often, on conjecture.

Two authors suggest that you stop guessing.

4.5.2   Rajczi and Meyer: Let the Subjects Decide

Alex Rajczi, a philosopher at Claremont McKenna, has proposed that you defer to subjects in deciding whether research is too risky. Instead of your IRB deciding if a protocol presents an acceptable mixture of risks and benefits, it would be deemed to do so if "some competent and informed subjects would agree to participate in it" (Rajczi 2004). Rajczi recognizes that subjects may have too little information to make a grounded decision about participation. However, "the fact that their choices are ungrounded does not mean that they are incompetent decision-makers. In fact, in a way they are *paradigm* decision-makers, because they are dealing with horrible uncertainty the only way a rational person can" (Rajczi 2004, emphasis in original).

Meyer urges us to put this idea into practice. She proposes that, for research involving competent adults, IRBs "cede the time-consuming and hopelessly subjective task of risk-benefit analysis to individual prospective participants. Each prospective participant would make an individualized decision about whether participation would be 'reasonable'—not in the abstract, but for her" (Meyer 2014, p. 323). IRBs would continue to supervise consent but would allow any informed and willing subject to participate in any research. In this open approach, some subjects, motivated by altruism, money, or their own reaction to a protocol's risks and benefits, would enroll in research that is more hazardous than would typically be approved today. IRBs would abandon paternalism, subjects would make their own choices, and more research would be conducted.

For all its appeal, this approach has two potentially fatal flaws. It leaves unaddressed the concern that the subjects who enroll might be foolish or gullible. Further, the regulations require you to conduct an evaluation of the risks and benefits of research and approve only research that is acceptable by this standard; you cannot simply pass the decision along to subjects. But there is a way to implement the Rajczi/Meyer suggestion.

4.6   Consent Before Approval

An administrative modification would permit you to give subjects more freedom of choice without abrogating your responsibility. This method, which is based on a hidden flexibility in the regulations, would allow you to be confident that subjects who enroll in relatively hazardous research do so with reasonable understanding.

The regulations require that your IRB approve the protocol and the consent form, but they do not specify the order. In practice, IRBs first approve the research, so the standard sequence is as follows:

1. The IRB approves the protocol and consent form.
2. The scientist enrolls subjects and begins the research.

Permission to Recruit but not to Begin. The modification would work as follows. Your IRB would review the protocol, conclude that it is too risky for many people, but recognize that some prospective subjects may weigh the risks and benefits differently from your committee. You would give the investigator permission to discuss the investigation with prospective subjects and obtain their consent, but not to begin the research.

If the investigator finds no willing subjects, the protocol fails Rajczi's test. If some subjects are recruited, that is useful information, perhaps enough for your IRB to permit the research to proceed. If your IRB is still hesitant, a committee member could discuss the protocol with the prospective subjects to get a sense of their level of understanding and voluntariness; your committee would then say yes or no. Even if you ultimately block the study, you will act with an understanding of how real people feel about it.

The modified sequence would thus be:

1. The IRB approves the consent form.
2. The scientist uses the consent form to enroll some subjects.
3. The IRB discusses the enrollment process with the investigator, meets with the subjects, or both.
4. The IRB decides whether or not to approve the protocol.
5. If the protocol is approved, the scientist begins the investigation.

To the best of my knowledge, no IRB has yet tried getting consent first and granting permission later. An IRB that does so should publish a description of its methods and results so that we can replace theory with experience.

Chapter 5
Consent in Biomedical Research

Consent, at its heart, is a *process*—an exchange of information capped by subject agreement. The form is not the consent (Lidz et al. 1988; Davis and Hurley 2014, p. 18). Nonetheless, IRBs pragmatically use the consent form as the primary tool to determine how subjects will be informed about a study. Consent honors subjects' right to choose and promotes their best interests as they define them.

5.1 Consent's Goals

Consent serves subjects. It notifies them that they are considering enrolling in an experiment, provides them with information they may use to make a decision about participation, informs them of what to expect if they enter the study, and enables them to accept or decline the risks of the research. *Consent serves society*: it permits research to be conducted by providing subjects who have accepted those risks.

The twin goals of consent are, thus, to enable subjects to enroll in research on their own terms and to permit research that will benefit us all. Consent does *not* funnel more subjects into research; it helps each person make the choice that is right for him or her.

5.2 Multisite Consent Forms

You should approach consent forms differently depending on their provenance.

© Springer International Publishing Switzerland 2016   47
S.N. Whitney, *Balanced Ethics Review*,
DOI 10.1007/978-3-319-20705-6_5

Your IRB has an ongoing relationship with local investigators and conducts their only ethical review; they can readily follow your instructions with regard to every detail of the consent form. Things are different for protocols that originate outside your institution and which may be conducted at dozens or hundreds of locations. The regulations, little changed since 1974, are modeled after a single IRB reviewing a protocol written by an investigator who will conduct the research locally; this approach is ill-suited to modern multisite research. In theory, local review might give each IRB a chance to adapt the protocol and the consent forms to the needs of the local community; in practice, local review adds no measurable benefit (Ravina et al. 2010).

For some multisite studies, your committee can rely on the review of another IRB (21 CFR 56.114, 45 CFR 46.114). When this is not the case—when you must conduct your own review—use a light touch if the protocol, and the consent form, have undergone ethics review elsewhere. When every IRB modifies a multisite consent form the result is often unethical cost and delay (Humphreys et al. 2003; Greene et al. 2006; Morahan et al. 2006; Ravina et al. 2010). If you find a glaring ethical problem you should respond appropriately, but please resist the temptation to tweak the consent form.

The rest of this chapter focuses on consent forms written by investigators at your own institution, where the cost of your intervention is lower and the potential benefit greater.

5.3 Presenting Risk and Benefit

Your IRB should ensure that the consent form presents the study's risks and benefits as accurately as possible. It should neither highlight a study's benefits and downplay its risks (Advisory Committee 1996, p. 452–454), nor exaggerate risks and understate benefits; either deprives prospective subjects of information they need.

Conservative and Unethical. It would be easy to behave cautiously, ensuring that risks are emphasized and benefits understated (Mazur 2007). This could even be seen as ethically obligatory, heeding Paul Ramsey's (Ramsey 1970, p. 10) admonition to scientists to lean against their natural inclination to deprive subjects of a balanced consent process (see Sect. 4.1.1). But for the IRB to manipulate estimates of risk and benefit toward greater caution would be to misapply Ramsey's suggestion. His advice was meant not for the committee but for scientists, who, in heeding it, lean away from their (biased) opinion and toward a position that feels conservative to them but is actually neutral.

In contrast, the IRB has no bias for or against the research, so it begins, and should remain, in a neutral position. A committee that leans against the research in the presentation of risks and benefits moves away from the accurate midpoint. Overestimating risks is not a conservative safeguard, it is an error.

Caffeine for Newborns. A study of the use of caffeine for premature babies illustrates how a consent form that exaggerates risk can impede subject choice.

In the early 2000s, some neonatologists routinely administered small doses of intravenous caffeine to premature infants in the belief that it improved their breathing; other doctors, worried that caffeine would cause more harm than good, never used it. This split in expert opinion made the time ripe for a trial, which was duly organized. In this study, every infant received routine care except that caffeine was administered based on random assignment rather than by local custom.

The consent form warned that an accidental overdose of caffeine had caused seizures. This is true, but the investigators took steps to control the rate of administration and prevent this complication, and the danger of an accidental overdose was far less than the respiratory complications that caffeine was meant to treat. Many parents nonetheless concluded that the study was hazardous and refused to enroll their babies. These parents also discussed with the doctors what routine care their infants should receive. In centers where caffeine had been in everyday use for years and the doctors were confident that it was helpful, most parents wanted their babies to receive it.

The absurd result was that parents were frightened at the possibility of their infant receiving caffeine in the trial but requested that it be given outside of the study. This inaccurate consent form delayed the evaluation of caffeine's effect and deprived babies, during the delay, of the benefit of this knowledge (Chalmers 2007).

Subject Rights. Finally, exaggerating risk and understating benefit could be seen as offering prospective subjects a margin of safety.

This may be one reason that Dennis Mazur and Jerry Menikoff emphasize the IRB's prudential duty to protect subjects from enrolling in research they might later regret (Menikoff and Richards 2006, p. 119; Mazur 2007). But some subjects might regret *not* participating, and all subjects deserve accurate information. To misstate either risk or benefit is to violate the Belmont Report principle of respect for persons.

5.4   Subject Understanding

The more potential subjects understand about research, the better. Ideally, they will become familiar enough with the investigation for their decision to reflect their individual values and preferences; in reality, not every subject grasps the details of the research this fully. The problem of imperfect subject understanding is central to your IRB's supervision of the consent process.

The FDA and OHRP gloss over this problem and the regulations ignore it entirely; but it is one thing to provide subjects with a detailed form and quite another for them to benefit from it. Today's consent forms, which may include dozens of pages of detailed material, often provide more information than subjects want or can use.

5.4.1   Less Is More

Scientists have long suspected that comprehensive consent forms do not serve subjects well. In 1969, pharmacologist Louis Lasagna collaborated with Lynn Epstein to study the effect of consent form length on subject understanding of the risks of a headache remedy. Subjects who read short forms had a surprisingly deficient grasp of the enumerated risks; those who read longer forms remembered even less. The longer the form, the less the understanding. Epstein and Lasagna concluded that "detailed descriptions of … side effects or toxic actions … apparently served to frighten the subject, who then was unable to classify the information usefully" (Epstein and Lasagna 1969). Their results overturned the belief that consent forms must include every risk, no matter how trivial or unlikely.

Federal regulators ignored this unwelcome finding; conscientious scientists did not, and called for research to find better methods (Fost 1979). In the years that followed, investigators in both clinical and research settings labored to develop forms that better inform, but progress has been slow (Candilis and Lidz 2010). A form (and sometimes supplementary techniques like an interactive DVD) may be a model of clarity, but not every subject wants to be, or can be, accurately and thoroughly informed. And even a form that appears clear may fail because we ask too much of it. Mark Hochhauser, a psychologist who specializes in readability, notes that "because consent forms are required to include so much detailed information, they create their own failure to inform. More information equals too much information, which creates memory overload, not more understanding." In summary: "Truly informed consent is impossible" (Hochhauser 2005).

Of course, your IRB should still do its best to help prospective subjects understand, as we will discuss in Sect. 5.5.

5.4.2 Ethical Considerations

A subject who does not fully understand research can still give ethically valid consent. People make many—or most—decisions in life without full understanding; there is no reason to require more in the context of research (Wertheimer 2011, p. 112–114).

Some authors do believe that complete understanding is an ethical requirement (Menikoff and Richards 2006, p. 119; Mazur 2007, p. 30; Amdur and Bankert 2011a, p. 175–176), but the original ethicists were too wise to demand the impossible. Paul Ramsey, a minister's son, wrote to an audience that included many doctors, "It is possible to analyze the motivations of normal volunteers so as to cast total doubt upon the freedom of their choice. But then one casts doubt as well upon most human decisions, such as the decision to become a physician or a minister. But a choice may be free and responsible despite the fact that it began in emotional bias one way rather than another, and consent can be informed without being encyclopedic" (Ramsey 1970, p. 3).

Franklin Miller and Alan Wertheimer believe that to require full understanding "is not only impossible and impractical but also unfair"

(Wertheimer and Miller 2008, p. 103). Wertheimer explains: "Somewhat ironically, a requirement of comprehension places a greater burden on *subjects* than they desire. A prospective subject will reasonably want an opportunity to comprehend, but may understandably resent being *required* to comprehend in part because it may be perfectly rational for a person to forego the acquisition of information or the effort to understand it" (Wertheimer 2011, p. 103, emphasis in original). Accordingly, scientists must disclose information, but subjects do not have to fully comprehend it for their consent to be morally transformative. Once a good faith effort has been made to inform subjects, in a manner your IRB has reviewed and approved, you can authorize the scientists to begin their morally important work.

5.5 Supervising Consent Form Writing

Your awareness of the ethics of subject understanding will not change what goes into the consent form—that is spelled out by the regulations—but it will enable you to structure the form so as to optimally promote subject understanding.

5.5.1 Helping the Investigator

You should try to provide such clear instructions that local investigators write forms that you can approve without changing a word.

Your institution may use research management software, in which the scientist answers a series of questions and the program populates a consent form. This process gives your committee peace of mind that every required element is included, and is especially useful for standard protocols like randomized controlled trials. This approach should be modified for other kinds of research, to avoid requiring every study to fit a Procrustean template.

Please provide investigators with as much information as possible about what answers are acceptable. Don't just ask "How will the data be secured?" If your standard is that a flash drive with protected health information must be encrypted, for instance, then say so.

Robin Penslar, a Canadian legal researcher, sensibly suggests that your IRB "distinguish between 'required' language and 'suggested' language. ... If the IRB has decided that only certain language is acceptable, say so and provide it as part of the application packet. ... If the IRB can provide suggested approaches to express various issues, provide several examples." Because no two studies are alike, you should indicate that you "will consider alternative language but that the examples provided have been determined to be acceptable ways to handle an issue. ... Do not try to force investigators to use specific language unless it truly is necessary" (Penslar 2006, p. 200).

5.5.2 Readability

Both the FDA and OHRP stipulate that the consent form must "be in language understandable to the subject or the representative" (21 CFR 50.20 and 45 CFR 46.116). Many IRBs therefore require forms to be written with a sixth- or eighth-grade readability score. This does little to improve subjects' ability to understand, for the underlying problem is not the difficult language but the complexity of the science (Hochhauser 2005; Ben-Shahar and Schneider 2014). Everyday language can give subjects a reasonable idea of what the study is about, but it is not always possible to fully explain complicated ideas in simple words. Your IRB should not require a specific readability level.

Rather than try to translate every concept in a scientific protocol into language that cannot sustain the informational burden, it makes more sense to structure the form so as to meet the needs of both elementary and advanced readers.

5.5.3 Format

The consent form's contents, including information that is not always germane, must follow the regulatory requirements. The regulations are not subject to negotiation; but they do give you flexibility in *how* this information is presented, and by an artful choice of sequence and format you can create consent forms that are more informative and therefore more ethical.

Sequence. Your institution's investigators should write consent forms that foreground the most important information (Smith 1999, p. 58–59; Baron 2006, p. 124; Davis and Hurley 2014, p. 19) and make it accessible to unsophisticated prospective subjects. An ideal consent form provides, in sequence:

1. A summary of the most important information that every subject should know, written, in deference to subjects who are not skilled readers, in the simplest possible language;
2. The most relevant additional information written in less elementary language;
3. Everything else that is relevant, for the rare information-avid subject; and, finally,
4. Irrelevant but required information.

Irrelevant Information. An ethically sound consent form contains only pertinent material; adding irrelevant information is unethical because it lengthens the form and competes with relevant material for subject attention. Nonetheless, if your IRB is typical, your consent forms include information that is of no real use to subjects. If the irrelevant material is there through force of habit, remove it. If it is required by institutional policy, the IRB chair should chat with the appropriate institutional official.

The irrelevant information is usually true; the question is whether subjects are likely to use it in deciding whether or not to enroll. A National Cancer Institute study of patients at risk for pancreatic cancer warns subjects that a blood draw may hurt: you may experience "a sharp pricking pain for just a moment when the needle goes into the vein in your arm" (National Cancer Institute 2011). This is true; it is also unhelpful and condescending.

There may remain an irreducible minimum of extraneous material, perhaps couched in legalese. Gather it all at the end of the form. The lawyer who demands its inclusion can hardly object if you label this section "important legal notices," even though few subjects will linger long over material with that title.

Foolishness. Try not to include anything that is ridiculous. When subjects read, for instance, that they won't be compensated should they be injured while completing a questionnaire, they will conclude that this is one of *those* forms that serve the institution's interests, not theirs. Don't encourage this train of thought.

Reviewing the Completed Form. As you review a consent form submitted by a local investigator for a local study, it does not matter if your template was followed precisely. You do need to make sure that the required elements are present and the consent form is a fair presentation of the research, its risks, and its benefits.

If there is a significant deficiency, follow Penslar's advice: "In most cases, it is unhelpful to say simply, 'The risks are not clear' or 'Include a statement about voluntariness.'" Instead, "tell the investigator exactly what you want, and where possible, provide the exact language you want to be used or give sufficient, well-worded instructions about the issue and options for handling it" (Penslar 2006, p. 201).

5.6   Editing the Consent Form

Let's assume the form before the committee contains the required elements in language that is typical for studies in your institution, including an accurate description of risks and benefits. Reading it through, you still see room for improvement. Should you edit it, require the investigator to do so, or leave it alone?

Some authors believe that IRBs have a duty to revise the consent form or to require the investigator to do so (Penslar 2006, p. 200; Mazur 2007, p. 80). Mazur has found that consent forms may need two or more revisions, because a first round of editing may reveal new issues that necessitate further changes (Mazur 2007, p. 80).

We can admire his commitment and still wonder if the added value of intensive editing repays the labor. No doubt some IRBs' edits improve subject understanding; others produce trivial changes or introduce errors (Burman et al. 2003). Robert Levine writes, "I believe that there is no more expensive or less competent redaction service available in the United States than that provided by an alarmingly large number of IRBs" (Levine 1986, p. 326). Ethicist Robert Amdur and educator Elizabeth Bankert provide this sage advice: "Resist the urge to make unimportant changes to the consent document. Every consent form can be improved with slightly different wording. … polishing and wordsmithing the document will not meaningfully improve the protection of research subjects" (Amdur and Bankert 2011b, p. 55). Eschew minor changes.

If your IRB now routinely edits consent forms, you should either restrict edits to egregious problems or study the editing process itself. How much time does it take? How different are the before and after consent forms? Would an outside observer, blinded to which form was first and which second, feel that the second was better?

The consent form is not a work of literature. It is a homely attempt to find common ground amid conflicting demands for comprehensiveness and clarity. It strives to show respect for the experimental subject while including every word of legal boilerplate. It will never be perfect, and if it meets the regulatory requirements and is reasonable that is good enough.

Chapter 6
The Social Sciences

Thus far we have focused on biomedical research, which is usually conducted in the medical school or hospital. In this chapter, we move down the street to the university.

IRBs have reviewed research in psychology since the system's founding; scholars in the other social sciences resisted ethics review with some initial success. But in 1995, as historian Zachary Schrag (Schrag 2010) has masterfully shown, federal officials mounted a covert campaign that forced universities to extend review to the other social sciences. As a result, many university IRBs routinely oversee work conducted throughout the social sciences, which present ethical issues quite distinct from those of biomedical research.

The humanities, like English and history, are even further from the concerns of the system's founders and the authority of the regulations. If your IRB chooses to oversee research in the humanities, you have fallen victim to the curse of power (see Sect. 3.2). If a higher institutional official requires you to do so, you are a victim of *their* power. This manual's advice on how to review the humanities consists of a single word: *don't*.

6.1 The Value of Dissent

If your IRB reviews research in the social sciences, you will have a ringside seat as scholars study fraught topics like racial and gender discrimination. You should interfere only when there is risk to subjects.

© Springer International Publishing Switzerland 2016
S.N. Whitney, *Balanced Ethics Review*,
DOI 10.1007/978-3-319-20705-6_6

Some authors disagree. Committee chair Jonathan Moss believes that the IRB has a duty to "forestall the public image problems and protect the institution's reputation by weeding out politically sensitive studies before they are approved" (Moss 2007). Joan Sieber and Martin Tolich caution that universities "are often called upon to explain why they sponsored or permitted research that has proven sensitive to public opinion. Your institution needs to be able to give a cogent and responsible explanation" (Sieber and Tolich 2013, p. 4).

The explanation is that our political system values dissent. During the student protests of the 1960s, law professor Harry Kalven, Jr. led a faculty group at the University of Chicago that studied "the University's role in political and social action." They concluded, "A university faithful to its mission will provide enduring challenges to social values, policies, practices, and institutions. By design and by effect, it is the institution which creates discontent with the existing social arrangements and proposes new ones. In brief, a good university, like Socrates, will be upsetting" (Kalven Committee 1967).

Citizens have a right to voice their opinions on the issues of the day; scholars have a right to study politically sensitive topics; and IRBs have a duty to approve research that will help ground public debate in evidence.

6.2   The Social Impact of Research

Your IRB has the power to hinder research whose results might support a particular political viewpoint about gun control, discrimination, or other charged topics. The regulations anticipate this possibility: "The IRB should not consider possible long-range effects of applying knowledge gained in the research (for example, the possible effects of the research on public policy) as among those research risks that fall within the purview of its responsibility" (45 CFR 46.111(a)(2)). OHRP notes that it is not part of the IRB's mandate "to evaluate policy issues such as how groups of persons or institutions, for example, might object to conducting a study because the possible results of the study might be disagreeable to them" (Office of the Secretary 2011). So, for instance, an IRB member who favors affirmative action should not block research that might show that such initiatives fail, just as a member who opposes affirmative action should not impede research capable of demonstrating a program's success.

Some IRBs nonetheless decide that some research is too volatile to permit (Klitzman 2013). Cornell psychologist Stephen Ceci demonstrated politically motivated ethics review in a troubling study in 1985. He found that IRBs often rejected research intended to prove that reverse discrimination had become a significant problem; one committee noted in alarm that an investigation "could set Affirmative Action back 20 years." But this was not merely liberal bias at work, for IRBs also objected to research intended to prove that discrimination is an ongoing problem (Ceci et al. 1985). In 2011, a blue ribbon panel led by epidemiologist and pediatrician Alan Fleischman confirmed that IRBs still delay or block "socially contentious research" and warned that this is unwise (Fleischman et al. 2011).

Fleishman, and the regulations, are right. You are responsible for the risks to subjects, not to society.

6.3 Freedom of Speech

There is an additional consideration when your IRB reviews research in controversial topics: censorship.

The Constitution and public policy provide unique protection for unpopular opinion, including dissenting academic and scientific speech. American scholars can therefore ask questions and pursue hypotheses that might elsewhere be forbidden as antisocial, and you may well review research that challenges social norms.

It is unconstitutional when someone acting on behalf of a state or federal government interferes with a person's "speech," an umbrella term for activities that include asking questions, recording the answers, and publishing an analysis of the exchange.

Consider an example. A journalist with an antisocial agenda can pose inflammatory questions to scientists about the genetic differences between people from Africa, Asia, and the Americas, and print the interview that results. A blogger can do the same, for the First Amendment protects everyone. What a journalist and blogger can do, a geneticist should be able to do as well. Yet at most institutions, an academic geneticist with an interest in social issues would have to get

IRB permission before interviewing his or her colleagues and publishing the results.

Let's assume that this takes place at a state university. If the IRB refuses to let the geneticist include pointed questions in the survey, could the scientist file suit against the committee for violating his or her constitutional rights?

Sieber and Tolich brush off the issue. In their view, journalism and academic scholarship differ "in the historical basis of their ethical mandates—the First Amendment versus the U.S. federal regulations of human research." Location matters: "Academic disciplines ... are situated within an academic institution ... while journalism is not." They conclude that "a journalist's ethical considerations originate as free speech found in the First Amendment ... Researchers do not have these same rights—end of story" (Sieber and Tolich 2013, p. 77, 79, 80).

This is not quite correct. Constitutional rights are not restricted to journalists; they extend to everyone, including the blogger and the geneticist, and the Constitution trumps any regulation.

Political scientist Ithiel de Sola Pool challenged "the new censorship of social science research" (Pool 1980). Pool's argument has been expanded by legal scholar Philip Hamburger, who believes that an IRB violates the Constitution when it regulates "inquiry, recording, talking, writing, and publishing." In his view, surveys and interviews are constitutionally protected speech (Hamburger 2007). Law professor James Weinstein disagrees, and he considers it far from certain that the Supreme Court would provide First Amendment protection for these activities (Weinstein 2007).

We do not have to resolve this debate. I suggest that you focus on the research's impact on the rights and welfare of subjects. If the research appears to be antisocial or immoral, that is not your problem, nor is it your place to act as a censor. Let it pass unmolested.

6.4 Psychology

Major concerns in the ethical oversight of research in psychology include deception and threats to subjects' self-esteem. Similar issues arise in sister sciences like economics, political science, and sociology.

6.4.1 Deception

Temporary deception is essential for some psychological research. For research in which people with full knowledge of the experimental plan could not serve as subjects, it is ethical to enroll subjects who do not know every experimental detail. The regulations accordingly permit your IRB to approve a consent procedure that omits some of the usual elements of consent provided that the research poses no more than minimal risk, the omission will not harm the subjects and is necessary for the research to be conducted, and subjects are debriefed afterward (45 CFR 46.116).

Social psychologist Elliot Aronson explains how debriefing works in practice. "Full disclosure is a vital part of our implicit contract with our subjects. Because no one enjoys being told that he has been duped, the disclosure must be done with tact and sensitivity, or the subject will feel that he or she has been a gullible fool. The experimenter can explain that because the cover story was so carefully crafted, just about *everyone* accepted it; far from being 'gullible,' the subjects behaved perfectly normally and reasonably." Aronson intends to "make sure that each and every one of our subjects leaves the experimental room with her self-esteem intact, in at least as good a shape as she was when she first came in, with the bonus of having learned something interesting" (Aronson 2010, p. 192, emphasis in original).

6.4.2 Threats to Self-Esteem

The most famous deceptive experiment was begun in 1961 by Yale psychologist Stanley Milgram. The trial of Nazi war criminal Adolf Eichmann had begun earlier that year. There was a lively debate over Eichmann's defense—typical of war criminals—that he was just following orders and therefore not ethically or criminally responsible for his actions.

The Experiment. Milgram wanted to see if ordinary people who are not citizens of a totalitarian state would follow unethical orders. The experiment was presented as an investigation in learning, and it required three people: a white-coated scientist, who acted as an authority figure; the subject, who was assigned to act as a teacher; and a learner, who was ostensibly also a subject, but was actually a member of the research team.

The "teacher" attempted to teach word pairs to the learner. When the learner, according to plan, did not learn, the teacher was instructed to flip a switch to administer an electric shock, which was initially slight but increased with each mistake. No punishment was actually delivered, but sound recordings gave the impression that the learner, who was out of sight in another room, was being shocked. As the simulated shocks became severe, the teacher heard the learner demanding that the experiment end. The white-coated scientist, however, urged the teacher to continue the experiment and increase the shocks as planned. It was up to the subject to obey—or refuse.

Many subjects went all the way to the maximum shock, 450 volts, which was described as very dangerous. They did not do so eagerly; almost all questioned the experiment and said they thought they should stop. "In a large number of cases the degree of tension reached extremes that are rarely seen in sociopsychological laboratory studies. Subjects were observed to sweat, tremble, stutter, bite their lips, groan, and dig their fingernails into their flesh. These were characteristic rather than exceptional responses to the experiment." Milgram recognized that he must debrief his subjects "to assure that the subject would leave the laboratory in a state of well being" (Milgram 1963).

Ethical Considerations. Developmental psychologist Diana Baumrind charged that Milgram had exposed his subjects to a risk of permanent harm; she also doubted his claim that debriefing prevented any injury (Baumrind 1964). Some scholars agree with her, others do not.

Elliot Aronson believes that Baumrind "overlooked the sturdiness and resilience of the average participant; even those who felt miserable about going all the way to the maximum level of shock later said they had learned a lesson of incalculable value. Not one of Milgram's subjects complained, and none reported having suffered any harm." Aronson was particularly impressed that, contrary to the harm that Baumrind assumed they would experience, Milgram's subjects felt they had benefited (Aronson 2010, p. 148–149). Sieber and Tolich also defend Milgram, pointing to "his great importance to an understanding of our moral failings as humans. He also teaches us (if we are paying attention) about the importance of learning how to stand up to unjust authority" (Sieber and Tolich 2013, p. 53).

Sieber and Tolich argue that Milgram's subjects' denial that they had suffered harm, their belief that they had benefited, and the value of the results indicate that the experiment was ethical. They suggest that with a fuller consent process, one that still withholds the details, it would be ethical to repeat the experiment today (Sieber and Tolich 2013, p. 53, 75, 143).

6.5 Surveys and Interviews

Your IRB is likely to review many survey and interview studies.

6.5.1 Risk and Benefit

The chief hazard of surveys and interviews is the inadvertent redisclosure of information that might lead to social or economic harm to subjects; you should therefore make sure that confidential data are secure. Other risks seldom merit attention. The evidence indicates that responding to questions, even on sensitive topics, is rarely hazardous enough to warrant your intervention.

Some authors nonetheless see significant risks in this kind of research. Dennis Mazur asserts that "questionnaire studies with the potential for serious consequences for participants would include studies involving persons with post-traumatic stress disorder or depression or persons who are victims of violence. ... a questionnaire study of post-traumatic stress disorder ... may elicit negative responses from the study participant that could include suicidal ideation or even suicide attempt" (Mazur 2007, p. 19, 56). Michelle Meyer believes that a survey or interview on a distressing topic could precipitate a panic attack and lead to "a cascade of psychological and economic harms" (Meyer 2014, p. 316). Neither Mazur nor Meyer provides a citation, or even an example. Yet their comments would justify an IRB that rejected research of this kind or imposed Mazur's study-killing recommendation that the investigator have counselors on tap to assist traumatized subjects (Mazur 2007, p. 56).

This cautious guidance is unsupported by the literature. A decade ago, mental health specialists Elena Newman and Danny Kaloupek reviewed the substantial empirical evidence on the hazards of surveys and interviews. There is some risk: "an appreciable subset of participants do express regret about participation, a proportion of whom also reports marked or unexpected distress. At this point, it is unknown whether such distress exceeds the range of minimal risk because we do not know whether or not these are new symptoms and whether or not the symptoms preexist but are intensified or sustained as a result of research participation." Yet "the majority of subjects who experience strong emotional reactions do not regret or negatively appraise their research participation. This confirms the suggestion that emotional distress can be understood as an indicator of emotional engagement with a research project rather than as a de facto indicator of harm" (Newman and Kaloupek 2004). In either the clinical or research context, insights may be upsetting, yet still sought after.

Eve Carlson is a scientist at the Veterans Affairs National Center for Post-traumatic Stress Disorder. Her group asked psychiatric inpatients to participate in an interview about post-traumatic stress disorder and childhood physical and sexual abuse. Thirty percent declined to participate—a reminder that prospective subjects can and do turn down research that might be upsetting. Of those who agreed to the interview, about 30 % were highly distressed. Nonetheless, among those who were the most upset, 37 % found the experience useful (Carlson et al. 2003).

Carlson asked her subjects why they found the interview upsetting and why they found it useful. The most common reason to find it upsetting was "remembering the past"; the most common reason to find it useful was that it "led to new insights" (Carlson et al. 2003). Sieber and Tolich comment, "Persons who are interviewed about a traumatic or stressful experience … typically report that they benefit emotionally from having a skilled interviewer listen to them; this helps them to clarify their own understandings of their experiences" (Sieber and Tolich 2013, p. 28). It is relevant that a research interview on a sensitive topic may be beneficial; but the main point is that while subjects may be upset, there is no reason to fear they will harmed.

6.5.2 *Modifications*

Mazur also urges IRBs to try to improve the wording of surveys and interviews. "The IRB must assess the hypothesis underlying the study and help the principal investigator develop the best questionnaire or survey that can be constructed to answer the questions of the study hypothesis. For example, if the questionnaire is asking participants for preferences, is it clear what is being asked? Can the IRB member sharpen the phrasing of the questions?"

This is sound advice only if your IRB is responsible for improving social science research in your institution. Otherwise, although you have the power to improve questionnaires, you should also have the judgment to refrain. There is nothing wrong with asking questions, so long as review is not prolonged, but you should not require an investigator to accept your suggestions.

6.6 Field Research

Some social scientists conduct field research, also called fieldwork. As the name implies, this is research in which scholars leave the laboratory and go into the community to discover, by observation or participation, how society functions. As they report their findings, social scientists join journalists, bloggers, pundits, and politicians in examining and commenting on people, communities, and cultures. Will van den Hoonaard, a Canadian sociologist with extensive ethics experience, has shown that the IRB should be at pains not to silence the scholar's voice in this public discussion (Van den Hoonaard 2002, 2011, 2016).

6.6.1 *Risk*

The chief hazards of field research include harm to reputation as a result of the indiscreet disclosure of fact or opinion. Risks like these are not your IRB's responsibility; no regulation can seal the lips of those who might embarrass themselves or others, nor should it try.

People are not hermetically sealed from the world. A member of a religious group can blog about his or her experience; an anthropologist who joins to learn about its customs can also blog, or can describe the community in a scholarly publication. The leader of a neo-Nazi group can distribute pamphlets about the evils of World Jewry; a sociologist who gains entrance to that group can describe the leader's behavior and beliefs in an article in the *American Sociological Review*. If members of the religious group, or the neo-Nazi leader, learn that a social scientist has profiled them in print, they may be infuriated or flattered, but their reaction to participant-observer research like this is not your IRB's responsibility.

6.6.2   The Sociologists' Dispute

If your IRB reviews field research, you should be aware that social scientists are engaged in a long-running internal dispute over its ethics, and in particular over how transparent and respectful the scholar should be toward its subjects. Some scientists favor an ethics of respect, others an ethics of inquiry.

Laura Stark's dissertation work is an uncontroversial example. Three IRBs let her attend meetings, take notes, and record their deliberations. In exchange, she protects their identities in her published work. She also—although this was probably not an explicit part of the agreement—presents their work with respect, even admiration (Stark 2006, 2012). Everyone wins.

There is a long line of social science fieldwork that is neither transparent nor respectful. In these studies, scholars, without revealing their identity or purpose, obtain entry to closed settings or groups. Social scientists have thus obtained an insider's view of apocalyptic religious cults, mental hospitals, juvenile gangs, Scientology, pentecostalists, extreme right-wing organizations, the police, the Ku Klux Klan, and marijuana dealers (Calvey 2008). This research, done without consent, enabled scholars to bring to academic, and sometimes public, attention information that their subjects may have wanted to keep private. Is this covert method ethical? Sociologists disagree.

What its practitioners term "covert," others call deceitful (Homan 1980; Davidson 2006). The American Sociological Association's *Code of Ethics* states flatly that sociologists "conduct their affairs in ways that inspire trust and confidence; they do not knowingly make statements that are false, misleading, or deceptive" (American Sociological Association 1999). British sociologist Roger Homan believes that covert research is not only deceptive, but that it also discriminates against the defenseless and powerless, harms its subjects, diminishes personal liberty, and betrays trust (Homan 1980, 1991, p. 96–126). This is the orthodox view, promoting an ethics of respect.

Dissident social scientists, who follow an ethics of inquiry, believe that it is less important to be respectful than to unflinchingly discover how people err and how society fails (Galliher 1973). Their work challenges established assumptions and sometimes intends to harm its subjects (Katz 2007; Feeley 2007). They celebrate sociology's willingness to expose evil organizations like the Ku Klux Klan.

Law professor James Lindgren points to the uselessness of social criticism that "must be so innocuous as never to cause anyone significant distress or harm" (Lindgren et al. 2007). Distinguished sociologist Howard Becker is more blunt: "A good study … will make somebody angry" (Becker 1970, p. 113).

Your IRB's Position. Your IRB has no reason to take sides in this controversy. You should treat all field research equally, whether the scholar follows an ethics of respect or an ethics of inquiry. You should not prevent the scholar from truthfully revealing the words and deeds of others, nor should you protect the corrupt, the brutal, and the racist from exposure. You are not the guardian of their secrets.

Sieber and Tolich disagree, and *Planning Ethically Responsible Research* is a comprehensive guide to respectful social investigation (Sieber and Tolich 2013). They intend their book to be used as a manual by both the social scientist who conducts research and the IRB that supervises it.

Sieber and Tolich are influential scholars, and they have every right to express their support for the ethics of respect among sociologists. Their advice to IRBs is a different matter. In my opinion, they do not explain why the ethical preferences of one group of social scientists should be imposed on the other under the authority of federal law.

6.7   Racial Discrimination

During the 1950s and 1960s, sociologists who studied racial discrimination were hobbled by a paucity of evidence. Apartment buildings might have no black tenants, for instance, but that did not prove discrimination; perhaps the landlords were telling the truth when they claimed that there happened to be no apartments available each time African Americans applied. The sociologists were skeptical but had no proof to the contrary.

This evidentiary dilemma was solved by a technique called discrimination auditing, in which matched pairs of white and minority researchers pose as apartment hunters or job seekers. Both testers apply (separately) for scores of (the same) apartments or jobs to see if they are shown an apartment or offered a job interview. Because the testers are very similar in every respect except race, responses that differ by race are presumptive evidence of discrimination. Of course, the landlords or employers are not informed that they are subjects in a study; that would vitiate the research.

In 1977, the Department of Housing and Urban Development used this powerful method to prove "persistent massive racial discrimination in housing" (Saltman 1979). This landmark result changed federal policy and provided crucial evidence in the struggle for equality. The courts understand that discrimination testing requires deception, but accept it as the only way to prove a violation of federal law.

Discrimination auditing continues to provide vital evidence about contemporary society. In the early 2000s, sociologist Devah Pager used pairs of matched testers (some white, some black) to apply for entry-level jobs in Milwaukee. Half of the testers, who were otherwise very similar, told employers they had a criminal record; half did not. In Pager's most striking finding, whites who had served time in prison were more likely to be invited for a job interview than blacks with a clean record (Pager 2003).

Research like this informs scholarly and public opinion without measurable risk. But Laura Stark has shown that some IRB chairs are unaware of the proud heritage of this testing method and confused about its ethics. She asked 18 chairs what their board would do with a protocol like Pager's. Stark omitted the variable of a prison record, and outlined a scenario in which white men and black men apply for the same job; the study would show if white applicants were called back more often than black applicants. Some chairs told Stark that they would approve the protocol; others viewed it as too hazardous to be approved.

One chair felt the study posed serious risks to a company that was found to be discriminating and to the university. What, she asked, if the investigator breached confidentiality and information about which businesses were discriminating became public? What if a company accused of discrimination sued the investigator and the university? Her board therefore would not approve the protocol without assurance that the firm, the investigator, and the university were all protected from this kind of harm—an impossible condition to meet (Stark 2012, p. 44).

The regulations define a "human subject" as a "living individual." Studying a company does not bring it to life or trigger federal protection on its behalf, nor should an IRB reject a study out of fear of possible litigation (see Sect. 3.2.3). I hope that if a protocol like this actually comes before this chair's committee, she would be willing to learn about the morality and value of discrimination auditing.

Research that abused racial minorities played a central role in the creation of the IRB system. If your committee has an opportunity to approve research that may ease the burden of a minority today, please take it.

Chapter 7
Biomedical Research Topics

We turn now to specific issues in biomedical research.

7.1 Archival Research

Not all biomedical research requires experimentation; some draws on data and specimens that are generated in ordinary medical care. Innovative surgeries and experimental drugs draw headlines, but sometimes a methodical scientist can save lives with only a stack of medical records and a telephone.

7.1.1 Cancer of the Vagina

Vaginal cancer was once a disease of older women. That changed abruptly in the 1960s, when teenagers began to develop an aggressive form of the disease. Many underwent radical surgery; many died (Herbst and Scully 1970; Herbst et al. 1979). Gynecologists, with no idea of the cause, were powerless to stem this murderous surge.

A team of Harvard doctors accepted the challenge. They studied the hospital charts of 8 adolescent patients and their mothers; they also examined the records of 34 controls—unaffected teenagers who were born at the same time in the same hospital—and their mothers. The scientists next contacted all 42 mothers and asked about their occupation, education, reproductive history, alcohol

© Springer International Publishing Switzerland 2016
S.N. Whitney, *Balanced Ethics Review*,
DOI 10.1007/978-3-319-20705-6_7

consumption, and much more. Two refused to cooperate; the other 40 provided every detail that was requested, as did the 39 daughters who were still alive.

This investigation predated the requirement for ethics review of research of this kind. If any of these women were upset that the scientists had reviewed their medical records, or that they had been called without first giving permission to be contacted, their reaction did not make it into the published report (Herbst et al. 1971).

The team's careful detective work produced a stunning result: diethylstilbestrol (DES), a hormone that had been given to reduce the chance of the mothers' miscarrying, had caused the cancers. Never before had a medication taken during pregnancy been shown to cause cancer in the child (Langmuir 1971).

Doctors no longer give DES to pregnant women at risk of miscarrying, and scientists no longer review medical records without consent.

7.1.2 Regulatory Oversight

Medical care generates copious amounts of clinical data and biological specimens. This material is accessed by many people besides doctors and nurses. Quality of care committees examine medical records and analyze lab or surgical specimens, coding specialists and insurance representatives use patient charts to generate charges and allocate financial responsibility, and law enforcement officials and inspectors from federal and state agencies examine patient records. All of these people routinely access this information without patient knowledge or consent.

And what of the scientist? The scientist must get permission.

This was not true when the IRB system was established. Early ethicists sought to suppress dangerous research conducted without consent. They paid little attention to research employing archival materials, with or without an interview to gain additional information—a set of epidemiological methods that can be called archival or health services research.

Once ethics review was in place, however, the curse of power (see Sect. 3.2) made it possible for IRBs to extend their scope to include researcher access to archival material. Then, in 2003, the Health Insurance Portability and Accountability Act (HIPAA) formally placed archival research under regulatory control. As a result, gatekeepers, including IRBs, were forced to make individual determinations about much health services research that was previously unencumbered.

When it is difficult or impossible to conduct archival research without consent, your IRB determines when consent may be waived, balancing the individual's desire for privacy and the public's need for the knowledge that research produces.

The chief risk of archival research is a breach of confidentiality, which could lead to personal medical information being revealed to an employer or insurance company. Data breaches do happen, as when a scientist's laptop is lost or stolen. If the research database includes subjects' social security numbers and credit card numbers, that is a security problem. But release of the medical information, resulting in loss of employment or insurability, can cause harm only if it finds its way to the employer or insurer, and there is no black market in stolen research data. When proper security measures are in place, the chance of a breach of confidentiality is small, the chance of the breach causing these harms is smaller still.

7.1.3 Ethical Considerations

People value both privacy and the benefits of research. Johns Hopkins scholars Lawrence Gostin and James Hodge suggest that policy should "seek to maximize privacy interests where they matter most to the individual and maximize communal interests where they are likely to achieve the greatest public good." They argue that it is ethical to use individual medical information without consent when "the potential for public benefit is high and the risk of harm to individuals is low. … Provided that the data are used only for the public good (e.g., research or public health), and the potential for harmful disclosures are negligible, there are good reasons for permitting data sharing" (Gostin and Hodge 2001).

The Belmont Report principle of respect for persons is sometimes invoked to argue that medical data should not be used without individual consent. But Case Western's Suzanne Rivera points out that the Report asks us to honor two other principles. "Beneficence suggests that uses of existing data and specimens should be maximized to derive the greatest amount of important knowledge possible. And justice requires a fair distribution of risks and benefits, encouraging broad participation in research across the population in exchange for information that will benefit everyone" (Rivera 2014, p. 253).

This approach is concordant with lay opinion. Ethicist Nancy Kass and her colleagues surveyed 602 patients and report that "when asked in the abstract whether they were willing to have their records used for research, without their knowledge or permission, the majority of our participants say no. Asking such a question in the abstract clearly seems negative to respondents, who perhaps see only the personal invasion without seeing any potential benefit." But when their subjects were assured that their privacy would be protected, "the overwhelming majority thought it was a good idea." Kass concludes that patients are interested "in supporting the research enterprise, provided safeguards are established to protect the privacy of their medical information" (Kass et al. 2003).

Because participation in archival research is essentially risk-free and can answer so many pressing questions about health and disease, many experts believe that subjects have a duty to allow their data to be used. The British scientists Richard Doll and Richard Peto write that "the right to medical care should, we suggest, generally continue to include the responsibility to allow the information gained in its course to be used for the benefit of others who develop a similar disease, or are at risk of developing it" (Doll and Peto 2001). Ruth Faden, Tom Beauchamp, and Nancy Kass, who helped create today's research ethics, make a similar argument, as we will see in Sect. 7.2 about the learning health care system.

7.1.4   The Common Rule

You may believe that subjects should allow their data to be used for archival research, but that does not give your IRB carte blanche to waive the requirement for consent. You must judge consent waivers on a case-by-case basis.

As your IRB makes these decisions, you probably follow two independent regulatory pathways. One is the Common Rule, which requires you to ensure "adequate provisions to protect the privacy of subjects and to maintain the confidentiality of data" (45 CFR 46.111(a)(7)). The other is the HIPAA Privacy Rule, which we will discuss in the next section.

The Common Rule states, "An IRB may approve a consent procedure which does not include, or which alters, some or all of the elements of informed consent set forth in this section, or waive the requirements to obtain informed consent provided the IRB finds and documents that:

1. The research involves no more than minimal risk to the subjects;
2. The waiver or alteration will not adversely affect the rights and welfare of the subjects;
3. The research could not practicably be carried out without the waiver or alteration; and
4. Whenever appropriate, the subjects will be provided with additional pertinent information after participation" (45 CFR 46.116(d)).

The critical step in applying this provision is determining when research cannot *practicably* be carried out without a waiver of consent. Mere inconvenience is not a justification, but if obtaining individual consent would add substantial time or cost, then obtaining consent, while possible, is impracticable. Similarly, if obtaining individual consent would significantly reduce the scientific value of the investigation, for instance by omitting data from people who cannot be reached, the research is impracticable and your IRB may waive the requirement for consent.

7.1.5 HIPAA

If your institution provides health care, the HIPAA Privacy Rule governs how you may use or disclose the protected health information (basically, medical records) that you generate. This section provides a simplified overview of key provisions of the Privacy Rule; for more details, see http://www.hhs.gov/ocr/privacy/hipaa/understanding/special/research/.

The Privacy Rule vests an institutional committee called the Privacy Board with authority to release health information without subject consent. While oversight of ethics and privacy may be separated, in many institutions the Institutional Review Board does double duty as a Privacy Board. If your committee serves in both capacities, you must follow the requirements of both the Common Rule and the Privacy Rule.

Some HIPAA provisions for the release of health information are mechanical and do not involve the Privacy Board/IRB at all:

- Subjects can always consent to the use of their information for research.
- If every (federally specified) identifier is removed from the dataset, it is termed "de-identified," is no longer considered protected health information, and may be shared with researchers.
- A "limited data set" is not fully de-identified and may be shared if the researcher signs a data use agreement stating that he or she will protect the information and use it properly.

Some investigations can be conducted under these provisions. But some research requires the retention of identifying information, like studies that link together records of the same individual from multiple datasets or of different but related individuals from the same dataset. The Harvard doctors could find the cause of vaginal cancer only by jointly analyzing the records of the mothers and daughters.

Waiving Consent under HIPAA. Your IRB, acting as a Privacy Board, steps in when a scientist needs information that includes identifiers and it is not practicable to obtain individual consent. The Privacy Rule, using conditions that are similar to the Common Rule, provides that you may waive consent if:

"(A) The use or disclosure of protected health information involves no more than a minimal risk to the privacy of individuals, based on, at least, the presence of the following elements;

   (1) An adequate plan to protect the identifiers from improper use and disclosure;

   (2) An adequate plan to destroy the identifiers at the earliest opportunity consistent with conduct of the research, unless there is a health or research justification for retaining the identifiers or such retention is otherwise required by law; and

(3) Adequate written assurances that the protected health information will not be reused or disclosed to any other person or entity, except as required by law, for authorized oversight of the research study, or for other research for which the use or disclosure of protected health information would be permitted by this subpart;

(B) The research could not practicably be conducted without the waiver or alteration; and

(C) The research could not practicably be conducted without access to and use of the protected health information" (45 CFR 164.512).

This, the key provision, is convoluted enough; but the Rule bristles with other stipulations. If your IRB acts as a privacy board, you need the counsel of someone who is intimately familiar with the Rule, either present in person or available by phone. Your board makes the judgment calls; the HIPAA expert makes sure that every box is checked.

A Flawed Regulation. As your IRB decides when to grant waivers of consent under HIPAA, you should bear in mind the sunny dreams of the Rule's drafters and the baleful impact it has had in practice. The drafters recognized that "severe limits on disclosures could do more harm than good" (Hamburg 2000). But in 2000, an HHS official reassured members of Congress that "the disclosures we propose to allow … are necessary for smooth operation of the health care system and for promoting key public goals such as research, public health, and law enforcement" (Hamburg 2000).

Most institutions were required to be compliant with the rule by 2003; its destructive effect was soon obvious (Institute of Medicine 2009, p. 4). Yet in 2015, an HHS website still quotes a 2007 document that states, "We do not believe that the Privacy Rule will hinder medical research. Indeed, patients and health plan members should be more willing to authorize disclosures of their information for research and to participate in research when they know their information is protected" (Office for Civil Rights 2007).

It is hard to know what to make of this statement. HHS's failure in 2000 to anticipate the impact of the Privacy Rule is unsurprising; those who draft regulations hope for the best. But we know now that the Rule has crippled health services research (Institute of Medicine 2009, p. 4).

HIPAA needs to be revised. In the meantime, your IRB can help the Rule function more nearly as it was intended. Authorize a waiver of consent when it would be impracticable to conduct the research without it.

7.2   The Learning Health Care System

In 1966, Henry Beecher showed that subjects in unethical experiments often thought they were getting routine clinical care (Beecher 1966). With Beecher's examples in mind, early ethicists viewed experimentation as inherently dangerous, and thus very different from ordinary clinical care (National Commission 1978; Miller 2006a). This made sense, since the research they had in mind involved interventions that would never be made in clinical practice, such as withholding needed treatment.

7.2.1   Integrating Research and Clinical Care

Archival research poses no such hazards, and the distinction between research and practice is irrelevant in investigations that analyze large-scale electronic archives. In time, scientists will use data from clinical care to help research and reciprocally feed research results back into routine care. This interplay, which eclipses the traditional distinction between clinical care and research, will accelerate as medical records become digitized. Ultimately, all of the electronic data captured in routine medical care will be used to evaluate and improve the care we all receive. Kass comments that in this system "practice is a continuous source of data for the production of generalizable knowledge, and the knowledge that is produced is used to continuously change and improve practice" (Kass et al. 2013), so the old emphasis on the research-treatment distinction is of diminishing value.

The Institute of Medicine has dubbed this exciting synthesis of treatment and research the *learning health care system* (IOM 2007, 2012). Each component—the aggregation of data, the analysis of databases, and more—is already being undertaken in limited ways. As data collection and analysis move to larger scales we will be able to achieve qualitatively superior results. Among its benefits, this new system promises to provide new ways to improve the health of racial minorities and the poor, with the prospect of reducing the health disparities that have long plagued us (Faden et al. 2013).

Some people are uneasy at the thought of researchers being able to routinely access their medical data. They may be reassured to learn that their individual information is of no interest to the scientists, who are usually looking for patterns that can be found only by extracting information from thousands or millions of records.

An example may help. Previous research showed that most patients who have had a heart attack benefit from taking a beta blocker, which is a medication that helps cardiac rhythm and workload; but beta blockers work better for some people than for others. Tomorrow's systems will be able to follow millions of heart attack patients and analyze the differences among patients. Does it matter, for instance, if the patient has rheumatoid arthritis, is African American, or was exposed to Agent Orange in Vietnam? If this large-scale data crunching shows greater or lesser benefit for specific groups, that information can be fed back into routine care, improving the health of the people whose data were used to answer the question.

7.2.2   Ethical Considerations

Hospitals have a legal obligation to collect and report data drawn from individual treatment records. This ongoing monitoring is central to measuring quality and reducing mortality; it would be unethical to do less.

What are the ethics of allowing academic scientists to access treatment data without individual consent? Privacy advocates argue that patients are morally entitled to control access to their data. Patients do have an interest in the privacy of their records, but it is not absolute, as we saw in Sect. 7.1.3. Faden, Kass, and colleagues have recently proposed that we rethink the individual's right to withhold data from the archival research of the learning health care system. They believe that patients "have an obligation to contribute to, participate in, and otherwise facilitate" research (Kass et al. 2013).

The idea that patients have a duty to participate in research is not new. I have mentioned Doll and Peto already; Mats Hansson, John

Harris, Rosamond Rhodes, and other scholars have long argued for the responsibility of individuals to assist low-risk investigations (Chadwick and Berg 2001; Doll and Peto 2001; Rhodes 2005; Harris 2005; Hansson 2010; Hansson et al. 2012). Faden's group adds a compelling argument for a fresh ethical approach.

7.2.3   Your IRB's Role

Once the learning health care system is fully in place, with ample notification to all patients that information from every clinical encounter is used to study current care and improve future practices, patients will have an affirmative obligation to allow their information to be used, and scientists will no longer need to seek permission to access patient data. But we are not there yet, for the learning health care system can become a reality only after today's regulatory barriers are dismantled. These new methods of archival research are bursting their regulatory bounds.

Congress needs to step in and establish a new system of oversight in which your IRB's duties will be dramatically different. Until that day, you should be aware of this evolving system, so that you can apply today's regulations with an awareness of where these changes in research and practice are leading.

7.3   Randomized Controlled Trials

Archival research is fast and frugal. This is the learning health care system's power: by analyzing mountains of data, it can show, for instance, a strong correlation between a particular treatment and lower mortality. But simply observing the outcomes of different patients given different treatments does not prove causality; the benefits of beta blockers for heart attack patients, for instance, were demonstrated by carefully controlled experiments. When scientists want to prove that an intervention saves lives, a randomized controlled trial is usually best.

Let's begin with a few definitions. A *trial* is an evaluation of an intervention, such as a new test or medication. A *controlled* trial compares one intervention to another, for instance a newer drug versus an older. One *arm*—one group of subjects—receives the experimental treatment, the other gets standard treatment and serves as the "control," hence, a *controlled* trial. A coin toss or equivalent method is usually used to assign subjects to arms at random—hence, a *randomized* controlled trial. The FDA requires randomized controlled trials for the evaluation of new drugs, devices, and biologics; OHRP oversees randomized controlled trials of many kinds.

In most controlled trials, the two interventions (medications, surgical procedures, etc.) produce roughly similar results. The relatively small expected difference is the ethical justification for conducting the trial, for the study should not be done if the scientists know that one treatment is significantly better.

Some trials raise thorny issues; (Miller 2010) they may, for instance, involve children or prisoners. This section focuses on trials in which subjects in both arms are free to choose.

Some trials are inappropriate for some patients, as when a doctor knows that one treatment is better for a particular patient or when a patient has a preference. But when experts cannot identify a better treatment for the average patient, a community doctor usually cannot identify a better treatment for an individual patient.

7.3.1 Risks Inside and Outside of a Trial

Most trials have risks that are little greater than the hazards of the underlying disease and its conventional treatment. Even when one arm offers a new and potentially better treatment, it is unusual for subjects in that arm to have dramatically better outcomes; when they do, monitoring committees ensure that the better treatment is soon available to every subject. In addition, subjects in both arms (probably) benefit by being cared for according to a carefully designed protocol.

This idea—that it is good to be in a trial—was once challenged on theoretical grounds. Law professor Charles Fried, in 1974, argued that patients who participate in research sacrifice the "good of personal care" because their treatment is controlled by a protocol and not by their own doctor (Fried 1974). Psychiatrist Charles Lidz carries this argument forward, listing the "risks and disadvantages" of participating in clinical trials, including "randomization, placebos, double-blind designs and restrictive protocols" (Lidz et al. 2004), and Jerry Menikoff asserts that trial participation is often a bad idea for a self-interested patient (Menikoff and Richards 2006, p. 119). All of these authors believe that patients would be wise to stay with their own doctor.

The evidence cuts the other way. Careful studies of how patients actually fare when they receive care from their own doctor, versus care in a clinical trial, suggest that they are better off in the trial (Vist et al. 2007). This may be particularly true for treatments that have not yet been thoroughly validated and may be available either inside or outside a trial. University of Texas scientist Jon Tyson explains why: a controlled study is "scrutinized not only by IRBs but also funding agencies, data-monitoring committees, peer reviewers, and the critical audience of physicians and scientists who read medical journals. This weighty net of supervision and monitoring is a potent incentive to investigators to use non-validated therapies in the safest and most effective way possible, on the basis of a careful assessment of the best available evidence" (Tyson 1995, p. 218–219).

John Lantos, pediatrician and ethicist, asks, "What if, instead of creating increased risk, clinical research creates increased benefit? Perhaps we should include, as part of the informed consent process for clinical research, a statement to the effect that participation in a research protocol has been shown to lead to better outcomes than nonparticipation" (Lantos 1999).

I don't see your IRB using language like this in a consent form any time soon. But it should help your deliberations to know that subjects inside a typical trial are likely to do at least as well as patients outside.

7.3.2 Nonphysical Risks

While many aspects of research participation are important, including time, expense, and freedom of choice, the benefits subjects care most about are health and life; the harms they fear most are disease and death. In general, medical interventions that promote subject welfare are ethical; harmful interventions are unethical. Discussions of trial participation therefore emphasize physical hazards. Law professor Richard Saver reminds us that research can also pose nonphysical risks, including "frustrated access to investigational technology, affront to dignitary interests, and participation in a study that fails to disseminate meaningful data in order to advance medical knowledge" (Saver 2006).

A research subject who is primarily concerned with disability and death might consider these nonphysical risks too nebulous to take seriously. But if there is a study in which your IRB feels that intangible hazards like these are significant, the consent form should disclose them so that subjects can take them into account.

7.4 Comparative Effectiveness Trials

The randomized controlled trial is a flexible template. One type of randomized study that your IRB is likely to review is a *comparative effectiveness trial* that compares two or more accepted interventions, like different ways of diagnosing, treating, or monitoring disease.

7.4.1 Identifying the Better Treatment

Before it approves a new drug, device, or biologic, the FDA requires proof that it is safe and effective, but not that it is better than other, already approved, treatments. Yet without such a comparison doctors do not know which treatment is best. Comparative effectiveness trials resolve this uncertainty.

One might think that archival research could play this role. If thousands of patients already receive each treatment, scientists might learn which is better simply by comparing the results. But the group with better outcomes might have been healthier to begin with or have another advantage; only random assignment makes the comparison reliable.

Consider, for example, the management of a heart rhythm disturbance for which the FDA has approved two drugs and one implantable cardiac device. A comparative effectiveness trial could use three arms, each with one of the competing treatments. Every subject would receive an FDA-approved treatment, and the result would be new information about which works best.

Because the interventions are already in clinical use, consent in a comparative effectiveness trial should reflect the reality that subjects encounter the same risks and benefits they would in clinical care (Tyson et al. 2014). Every subject in a comparative effectiveness trial must consent to the risks and benefits of the specific intervention he or she is assigned to, for instance the drug or the device. Your IRB must decide what consent is ethically required for random assignment itself. The conventional answer is that subjects must also consent to randomization, which makes good sense for a study, like the cardiac arrhythmia trial, that compares a pill and a procedure. But sometimes the interventions are so similar that patients are unlikely to have a preference (Eisenberg 1977).

7.4.2 Faden's Bold Ethical Proposal

Faden, writing with Beauchamp and Kass, believes that subjects might ethically be enrolled in some comparative effectiveness trials without consent, at least as consent is understood today. She assumes that these studies are conducted in a clinic or hospital that is part of the learning health care system, where patients accept that research is part of daily practice. Such a system is ethical, in part, if it has "core commitments to engagement, transparency, and accountability in ways that are keenly sensitive to the rights and interests of patients" (Faden et al. 2014). Here patients help set the priorities for comparative effectiveness trials and participate in their ethical review.

I would describe this active involvement of patient representatives, and transparency of the research enterprise, as constituting a substitute for informed consent for carefully selected studies. In this setting, a low risk randomized trial might require no consent; Faden's example is of a common condition in which some clinicians order a laboratory test once and others order it twice. Similarly, a randomized trial comparing the effectiveness of two very similar medications might entail at most only a rapid, oral consent (Faden et al. 2014).

Ethics will still often demand full consent. Research with greater risk or in which subject preferences are likely to play an important role, like a study that compared a medication to an implantable cardiac device, would require conventional consent.

7.4.3   Waiver of Consent in Special Circumstances

In each of these examples, conventional consent is practicable; other circumstances might require a different ethical solution. Consider, for instance, research in which time is short.

The SUPPORT trial was an 18-center study of the breathing and health of extremely premature babies. It is also an important example of the challenges of contemporary ethics review and federal oversight; we will refer to it repeatedly.

One branch of the study compared two well-accepted methods of respiratory assistance just after birth. In order to conduct this research with consent, the scientists had to approach several expectant mothers for everyone who delivered an eligible infant. Obtaining consent cost 2 years and $200,000; it also produced a distorted enrollment that underrepresented the most vulnerable infants (Rich et al. 2010, 2012).

Since both treatments were already in common use, SUPPORT was a comparative effectiveness trial (Wootton et al. 2013). Faden's approach could be adapted to conduct the SUPPORT study without consent as follows:

- The community would be informed that research to improve newborn care is being conducted—with consent when practicable and without consent, after the approval of community representatives, when impracticable
- Every patient in the hospital would be notified of this practice, and given an opportunity to learn what studies are ongoing
- Members of the community would be involved in the decision to implement the SUPPORT study
- Parents of infants enrolled without consent would be notified as soon as possible

This approach would be cheaper and scientifically better than getting consent from every mother before delivery. It would also be morally superior: it is of greater ethical value to include the most vulnerable babies in the research than to require their mothers to consent to interventions routinely provided without consent in ordinary care (Whitney 2012).

John Lantos and John Spertus, and the editors of the *New England Journal of Medicine*, have argued that consent to comparative effectiveness trials like SUPPORT should reflect the reality that research like this imposes no risks above those present in ordinary clinical care

(Lantos and Spertus 2014; Editors 2014). In theory, IRBs could have waived consent in the SUPPORT study under the Common Rule on the grounds that delay, cost, and distorted enrollment otherwise rendered the study impracticable. But for now your IRB must hew to conventional practice, since OHRP has made it clear that it expects comparative trials to be conducted only with an exhaustive consent process (Office for Human 2014).

The regulatory climate is not yet right for comparative effectiveness trials to be conducted without consent, but Faden is surely right that we must move in that direction.

7.5 Justice

Justice is the ethical foundation of democracy. The moral philosopher John Rawls begins *A Theory of Justice* with the words, "Justice is the first virtue of social institutions, as truth is of systems of thought. ... Each person possesses an inviolability founded on justice that even the welfare of society as a whole cannot override" (Rawls 1999, p. 3).

7.5.1 Unjust Burdens

The Belmont Report points to the injustice that occurs when one group reaps the benefit of research while another group, such as the Tuskegee syphilis study subjects or poor ward patients, bears its burdens (National Commission 1978). Today, some research is specifically designed to decrease health disparities, and poor people who enroll in research are often paid. But injustices remain important even though they are less common.

The Report cautions that "some classes (e.g. welfare patients, particular racial and ethnic minorities, or persons confined to institutions)" should not be "systematically selected simply because of their easy availability, their compromised position, or their manipulability." Your IRB should act when it identifies a problematic distribution of burdens and benefits. This topic is discussed more fully in Sect. 7.6 about vulnerable groups.

It is easier to identify groups that are being exploited than to ensure that the benefits of research are distributed fairly. The Report slips when it urges that "whenever research supported by public funds leads to the development of therapeutic devices and procedures, justice demands … that these not provide advantages only to those who can afford them" (National Commission 1978). It is hard to see how you could heed this admonition. By definition, any new treatment will benefit only those who can afford it.

7.5.2 The Governmental Pursuit of Justice

Congress and the funding agencies pursue justice as they distribute billions of federal research dollars. NIH, for instance, seeks advice from scientists, patient organizations, an advisory committee, and the NIH director's Council of Public Representatives; it then funds projects that address our most pressing needs.

Justice is at the forefront of these decisions, which prioritize diseases that impose the greatest burden of suffering and critical problems like racial health disparities. Senior federal officials implement these priorities as they allocate funds to thousands of specific projects. Your IRB promotes justice every time it approves a protocol that is part of this comprehensive program.

Your IRB should not modify or disapprove individual protocols in an attempt to serve justice unless you are unusually well-informed about the overall federal plan. You review research one protocol at a time, and any single study is only one of the many strands of our pursuit of justice.

Klitzman illustrates the point. He interviewed an IRB chair who felt that a protocol that required subjects to have high-speed internet access would unfairly exclude the disadvantaged. For the program to continue, the IRB required the scientists to provide temporary internet access for prospective subjects who were without it (Klitzman 2013).

The goal of narrowing the gap between the digital haves and have-nots is well intentioned but not well informed, for the fundamental question is whether federally funded research, taken in its entirety, adequately addresses the health needs of people who are not routine internet users. It is a rare IRB that will know the answer or be able to improve the government's efforts to ensure justice.

7.5.3   The Private Pursuit of Justice

IRBs review research funded by pharmaceutical companies and non-profit groups like the American Heart Association. These organizations, as private actors, are not responsible for advancing justice. Pharmaceutical research may produce either a breakthrough drug or a me-too medicine that offers little added benefit; but while trivial research is a cause for concern, it is outside the Belmont Report's conception of justice, and it should be outside yours as well. Your IRB is not in a position to judge a company's research priorities or reallocate its resources. You have the power to block their intended use, but you should resist that temptation. Your IRB should protect subjects' rights and welfare and let funders decide how to spend their money.

7.6   The Vulnerable

Some groups, such as children, prisoners, and mentally disabled persons, are handicapped in their efforts to seize opportunity and avoid peril. For the vulnerable, as for us all, ethics considers both risk and benefit. As Charles Weijer writes, "Justice fully understood requires that a balance be struck between protecting the vulnerable sick from burdensome research and allowing their inclusion in potentially beneficial research" (Weijer 1999).

7.6.1   Regulatory Overprotection

The regulations focus on protection. OHRP requires your IRB to ensure that "when some or all of the subjects are likely to be vulnerable to coercion or undue influence, such as children, prisoners, pregnant women, mentally disabled persons, or economically or educationally disadvantaged persons, additional safeguards have been included in the study to protect the rights and welfare of these subjects;" FDA has a similar requirement (45 CFR 46.111(7)(b) and 21 CFR 56.111(7)(b)). Since the enumerated groups are only examples, your IRB can define any group as vulnerable and take any measure you see fit to protect it. This grant of power to your IRB is a reaction to research that abused defenseless groups, like the African-American sharecroppers of Tuskegee and the patients at the Jewish Chronic Disease Hospital (see Sect. 2.3).

Some groups are as vulnerable today as ever, but their situation with regard to research has changed. Today's regulations protect all subjects, vulnerable or not, by ensuring that the risks and benefits of research are reasonable and that the consent process is appropriate. These requirements would have thwarted the unethical studies that Beecher denounced, whether or not the subjects were in a vulnerable group. As a result, the requirement that you take special steps to protect the vulnerable, aimed at yesterday's scandals, is redundant; it demands that you provide "additional safeguards" without explaining why today's universal protection is inadequate or how you should augment it. There is, unsurprisingly, a dearth of published examples of IRBs that identified a vulnerable group, enacted an additional safeguard, and demonstrated that the group was thereby better off.

Your IRB cannot change this archaic regulatory requirement, but you can be judicious when you consider requiring additional safeguards; this will reflect the new reality that much research imposes no net harm (like comparative effectiveness trials), is without harm (like survey and interview studies), or offers a chance of benefit (like the early trials of new AIDS drugs).

7.6.2   Fighting Health Disparities

Philosopher Baruch Brody summarizes the transformation in how we see research with the vulnerable: "The older conceptualization, the protective conception, emphasized the protection of vulnerable subjects from being used without their consent and from being exploited in excessively risky research. The newer conceptualization, the balancing conception, incorporates access to the benefits of research as an additional demand of justice. As a result, justice in research is now seen as demanding a proper balance of access to the benefits of research with protection from unconsented use and from exploitation" (Brody 1998, p. 32).

When, under the guise of protection, the vulnerable are kept from research like comparative effectiveness trials that presents no net harm, vulnerable individuals do not benefit and vulnerable groups are harmed.

African Americans, for example, have the highest combined cancer mortality rate of any group (Ward et al. 2004) and an infant mortality rate that is approximately double that of whites (Mathews and MacDorman 2011). Latinas receive less prenatal care, fewer mammograms, and are given less adequate pain medication for cancer (Fiscella et al. 2000). Only by including minorities and other vulnerable individuals in research will the treatment that is developed reflect their needs. Your IRB should be cognizant of the importance of health disparities and permit scientists to enroll vulnerable subjects in low risk studies.

The SUPPORT trial, which is introduced in Sect. 7.4.3, is a good example. At the time of the study, the recommended range of oxygen for premature babies was broad. Every infant in the trial received oxygen within that range; the level was varied in an attempt to find the ideal amount. Because every baby received an oxygen level that met the standard of care, inclusion in the trial imposed no risk beyond the hazards of prematurity itself.

Since prematurity and infant mortality burden poor minorities more than affluent whites, the trial should have included a modified consent process to ensure appropriate inclusion of the minority poor. Understandably, however, all concerned assumed that OHRP would require a comprehensive, conventional consent process, no matter the cost in time, money, and distorted enrollment. When the results were tallied, one group was underrepresented: the babies of minority women with no health insurance and limited education—a precise echo of the regulation's concern about the "economically or educationally disadvantaged" (Rich et al. 2010, 2012; Whitney 2012).

The IRB system deserves credit for helping extinguish research that abused the vulnerable, and vulnerable subjects sometimes still need to be protected from hazardous research. But for research that is no riskier than ordinary clinical care, your IRB should facilitate the enrollment of vulnerable groups.

7.7 Paying Subjects

Some subjects are paid. Subject payments serve, as Christine Grady says, both as "a sign of respect for the contributions of research subjects and a way to facilitate valuable research" (Grady 2005).

The NIH's original IRB, the Clinical Research Committee, was not troubled that some of the Clinical Center's subjects were paid. The 1966 guidelines that established the IRB system did not mention subject payment, nor does the Common Rule. This is appropriate, for paying subjects usually creates no ethical problems.

7.7.1 Respecting Subject Choice

People participate in research to get better care, to help others, to be paid, and for other reasons; none is morally suspect and none should attract undue IRB attention. You could micromanage subject payment, but that doesn't mean you should. If a subject who has been properly informed wants to get better care, to help others, or to make money, that is not an ethical predicament; it is how people make decisions. Your IRB should usually permit scientists to offer more money to persuade more prospective subjects to enroll.

"The point of the idea of autonomy," writes psychologist Jonathan Baron, "is that people should be able to choose what is best for them according to their own values. If people value money so much that sufficient amounts of money will induce them to do something, that is one of their values. They think they are better off taking the money. Unless we have good reason to think they are wrong, we should take their word for it." If subjects are paid to participate in commercial drug or medical device testing, they "think they are better off with the money, and it is very likely that they are. So, if the subjects are better off, if the companies and their stockholders are better off, and if future patients are better off, this is a win-win-win proposition" (Baron 2006, p. 157).

The only cause for concern would be a payment plan that unfairly penalizes subjects who withdraw. It is acceptable for the investigator to pay a bonus to subjects who complete the project. But for research in which subjects might have a compelling reason to drop out, like side effects from an experimental treatment, it would be wrong to withhold all payment from subjects who withdraw.

Lotteries. Some investigators with limited budgets offer participation in a lottery as a reward for participation. One author is concerned that "lotteries violate the principle of justice because of the unequal distribution of something of value—namely, that only one person wins the lottery" (Gordon et al. 2011, p. 123). That's the (ethically unproblematic) point: one person collects a significant reward rather than many receiving a pittance.

7.7.2 Coercion

Some authors worry that paying subjects may be a form of coercion or a violation of the principle of justice. The FDA, whose regulations in this area diverge from the Common Rule, instructs IRBs to "review both the amount of payment and the proposed method and timing of disbursement to assure that neither are coercive or present undue influence" (Food and Drug Administration 2014).

Menikoff deftly dispatches the question of coercion. "In general, offering someone an additional opportunity to earn some money is not the sort of thing we view as being coercive. Coercion more typically takes place when someone threatens to do something bad to you unless you do the desired act: 'Pay us the million dollars or your kidnapped daughter gets killed.'" A subject who is offered money to enroll is in a different situation. "Creating an additional opportunity that we can choose to accept or reject is not commonly thought of as coercive. The fact that it is an exceptionally good opportunity—that we might get paid a lot more than we were expecting—probably just means that it is our lucky day, not that we are being coerced" (Menikoff and Richards 2006, p. 216). Offering payment does not coerce anyone to participate; it only rewards them if they do.

Payment and the Poor. A scientist who wants more subjects, like a shopkeeper who wants more employees, can raise the proffered compensation until enough people accept.

Paying subjects to participate in research could lead to the disproportionate enrollment of poor people. Would this violate the Belmont Report principle of justice? The Report urges us to reject past practice in which "the burdens of serving as research subjects fell largely upon poor ward patients, while the benefits of improved medical care flowed primarily to private patients" (National Commission 1978).

Times have changed. Those "poor ward patients" were usually offered neither choice nor payment; poor patients today enroll voluntarily and some do so for the money. The more they are paid, the less their enrollment offends our love of justice.

7.7.3   Setting a Cap on Wages

Cardiologist Neal Dickert and ethicist Christine Grady, in a thought-ful exploration of the arguments for and against different models of subject payment, are uneasy about allowing the market to set the price of a research subject's participation. They recommend instead a planned-wage system in which subjects are paid a standardized amount that would be the same "both among different protocols and between research and other forms of unskilled labor." This would avoid some subjects being paid more than others. Uneven payment, they argue, would violate the ethical principle that "similar people should be treated similarly," so a set wage better embodies the prin-ciple of justice (Dickert and Grady 1999).

Menikoff's rebuttal is tart. "It is ironic indeed that, in pursuit of 'justice,' we might continue to pay poor people amounts that seri-ously undervalue the contribution they make to society when they participate in research studies. Somehow, that policy seems more *un*just than just" (Menikoff and Richards 2006, p. 221, emphasis in original). Alan Wertheimer and Franklin Miller observe that ethical commentary is too often "parochial" and is typically "not tested by examining comparable situations in other domains of human affairs" (Wertheimer and Miller 2008).

We can apply their suggestion by viewing a cap on research sub-ject wages in the light of similar initiatives in the larger economy. Our society roundly rejects the idea that government should set a cap on the wage an employee can earn or the price a shopkeeper can charge. Central planners have tried to set maximum wages or prices many times, including the French Revolution, the Soviet Union, the 1971–73 American price controls, and New Zealand's 1982 freeze on wages, prices, and interest rates; neither Robespierre, Khrushchev, Nixon, nor Muldoon could sustain them. Central planning doesn't work; the market does.

7.8   Emergency Research

Your IRB always expects to see an appropriate consent process in place. A motorist who suffers a concussion, for instance, must con-sent before being enrolled in a trial of post-concussion surveillance.

But what of accident victims who are unconscious because of a severe—potentially fatal—head injury? They cannot consent, and the therapeutic window for an intervention is usually too short to obtain consent from a proxy. Patients with conditions like severe stroke, prolonged seizures, and (obviously) sudden death, are similarly unable to consent. In this discussion, I assume that consent, by subject or proxy, cannot be obtained because of the nature of the emergency.

7.8.1   Criteria for Approval

An IRB may approve research without consent in emergency conditions like these if the relevant regulatory conditions, summarized here, are met:

- The IRB must determine that:
  - Potential subjects are in a life-threatening condition,
  - Available treatments are unproven or unsatisfactory,
  - Risks and benefits are reasonable,
  - Informed consent is not feasible, and
  - The research offers the prospect of direct benefit.
- The IRB must ensure that provisions are made to obtain the consent or refusal of subject or surrogate when that can be done:
  - Prior consent of the subject or surrogate is preferred if possible,
  - Otherwise subject or surrogate must be informed as soon as possible and given an opportunity to withdraw.
- The IRB must ensure that additional protections are provided:
  - The community must be consulted,
  - There must be an independent data monitoring committee, and
  - The community must be informed of the results after study completion.

For the full details, see the FDA and HHS regulations (21 CFR 50.24 and 61 Federal Register 51531).

The regulations require your IRB to approve a method for the "community" to be consulted. The community could be, for instance, people who live within a specific catchment area or patients with a condition that predisposes them to an emergency complication. Consulting the community, in practice, means that the scientist (or the IRB) informs members of the community about the proposed research and invites feedback. The regulations require no specific process, so your IRB is free to accept any method that gives some of the people who might be affected by the research an opportunity to be informed and respond.

7.8.2   Ethical Considerations

If *treatment* in emergency conditions is to be given, it must be without consent. This is not an ethical problem—we have no choice. If *research* in emergency conditions is to be conducted, it must also be without consent. But some commentators believe that consent in research is morally obligatory; in their view, research without consent can never be ethical (Katz 1997; Capron 2014, p. 147).

This perspective has an honorable lineage that dates back to the Nuremberg Code, which emphasized that the consent of the subject is "absolutely essential" (Nuremberg Code 1947). But physician and ethicist Norman Fost argues against the rigid application of this maxim. "Informed consent is not an end in itself. It is a means, an instrument designed to achieve the end of protecting patients from harm and protecting their right to self-determination." The unconscious patient must trust the doctor to act in his best interest, but for unproven emergency interventions, the doctor does not know what treatment is best. When the doctor can offer no proven intervention, Fost argues, it is as acceptable to administer treatment as part of a controlled trial as to use a treatment, not part of the trial, that has never been proven to be effective (Fost 1998).

The evidence base for ordinary clinical practice is surprisingly sparse; as pediatrician Susan Wootton comments, "most treatment methods have never been rigorously assessed to ensure their risks do not exceed their benefits" (Wootton et al. 2013). For emergency conditions in particular, doctors often use treatments that have never been proven to be better than other interventions, or even better than nothing at all.

Any of us could be either a subject in emergency research or a beneficiary of the knowledge gained. Jonathan Baron therefore invokes Rawls's veil of ignorance, as follows:

- If you suffer a cardiac arrest or a severe head injury, you do not know in advance (this is the "veil") if you will be a patient or a subject in a study of your medical problem
- Some emergency departments study new interventions; some do not
- Only interventions that offer the prospect of direct benefit for your problem can be studied

Given these conditions, would you rather be taken to an emergency department that investigates new treatments or one that does not? (Baron 2006, p. 108)

Iain Chalmers goes one step further to argue that it is unethical *not* to conduct research in emergency conditions, and urges us to routinely study unproven practices so that we may embrace the effective and discard the destructive. As an example, Chalmers cites the use of steroids in patients with severe head injuries. Steroids were, for years, the standard of care—until a trial that enrolled thousands of unconscious subjects showed that those who were given steroids were more likely to die than those given a placebo (Edwards et al. 2005; Chalmers 2007). This lifesaving research could be done only with a waiver of consent.

7.9 Phase 1 Cancer Trials

When animal research suggests that a new anticancer agent has promise, it is cautiously tested in small phase 1 trials, so named because they are the first phase of drug evaluation in humans. Patients are eligible only if they have failed any conventional therapy and are expected to die.

Some authors believe that patients should be told that Phase 1 trials are intended to assess drug toxicity, not benefit, and that the chance of benefit is minuscule. These authors fear that consent forms do not accurately convey the reality of trial participation, allowing subjects to harbor unrealistic hopes for benefit (Horng et al. 2002; Menikoff and Richards 2006, p. 118–119; Miller 2006b). In their view, when patients enter these studies the winner is the investigator, who adds another study to his publication list; the loser is the subject, who signed up in hopes of personal benefit but will more likely experience toxicity and dashed hopes.

Fortunately, the reality is less dire.

A Reasonable Chance of Benefit. Phase 1 trials are used to determine the maximum tolerated dose of a new medication, which will then be used in later, larger studies to measure benefit. These initial trials are too small to show how effective a new agent is for any particular cancer. But seeing if the drug produces some benefit is an important goal (Arkenau et al. 2008), since a drug that shows no benefit is unlikely to be studied further (Han et al. 2003).

Today's trials offer a modest but real chance of benefit. Oncologist Maurie Markman observes that recent phase 1 trial results "are quite comparable to that anticipated for many current programs routinely utilized as 'standard-of-care' in the treatment of advanced and metastatic malignancies. ... Based on increasingly solid data, it is reasonable to conclude that future proclamations of the fundamental absence of therapeutic intent associated with phase 1 antineoplastic drug trials simply do not reflect the current reality of cancer drug development" (Markman 2008).

The assumption that patients are likely to experience severe toxicity is also unfounded, in part because newer generations of therapy, sometimes called molecularly targeted or biological agents, are often relatively benign. Older cytotoxic agents (conventional chemotherapeutic drugs) attack all rapidly dividing cells—those in normal bone marrow and digestive tract as well as those in a tumor. Biological agents are generally less toxic because they target a molecular process or structure that is more specific to cancer (Arkenau et al. 2008).

Leaving the Door Open for Hope. The other major ethical concern is that even an accurate consent form may encourage false hope. How, then, should consent forms present risk and benefit? I would consider it reasonable to say, for instance, that there is a small chance of benefit, as well as a significant chance of toxicity, with death from the experimental medication occurring in about one patient in 200.

This is not gloomy enough for some commentators; one believes that consent forms should say, "Based on prior experience, the chance that you will feel better or live longer as a result of participating in this study is almost zero" (Miller 2006b, p. 462). Jerry Menikoff is concerned that overoptimistic forms encourage "delusional thinking" in subjects who enroll (Menikoff and Richards 2006, p. 119).

That is his opinion; but it's not clear that people who enroll in phase 1 trials are deluded. Someone who has no treatment options is not obviously foolish to choose a trial that offers a small chance of modest benefit (Wertheimer 2011, p. 9). Further, the decision to join a trial need not rest on a mathematical weighing of the odds. Insightful psychiatrist Kevin Weinfurt has found that subjects sometimes feel a "moral imperative" to live in hope instead of fear (Weinfurt et al. 2008). This desire is anything but delusional.

A Subject's Perspective. In June, 2014, Susan Gubar (Gubar 2014) wrote, "When I signed up for this clinical trial of a medication never before used on human beings, I was informed that Phase 1 studies do not extend life. They are designed to test dosage and toxicity. Since August 2012, however, the pills, as yet unnamed, have been keeping my recurrent ovarian cancer at bay." While on the trial, she has experienced "one daughter's wedding, the birth of a grandson, a family reunion, the return to town of a stepdaughter, and the writing of this blog. With no illusions about a cure, I nevertheless marvel that I have the strength to make the bed without collapsing between the top and bottom sheets."

Gubar has an impermanent reprieve that oncologists call a "response." Of course, patients don't want a reprieve; they want to be cured. No phase 1 trial consent form should suggest that a cure might result; the possibility is too remote. But in most patients, hope for cure coexists with a less-focused hopefulness that something good may come of the present circumstances (Whitney et al. 2008). We can be honest with phase 1 trial subjects without crushing their desire to live in hope.

Chapter 8
FDA and OHRP

The FDA and OHRP control the IRB system; if your IRB reviews a variety of biomedical protocols, it functions under the watchful eye of both. If you understand their position in our political system, it will be easier to keep in their good graces.

8.1 Agencies Under Pressure

Both agencies are superbly positioned to facilitate research to promote the public welfare. The FDA knows the public is eager for new treatments for conditions ranging from prematurity to Parkinson's disease. Officials at OHRP have access to data on the health of the American people, including areas of particular moral concern, such as the disparities in health between rich and poor, white and black. But neither agency makes the most of its position. For the FDA and OHRP, as for most federal agencies, inaction is safer than action, even when doing nothing is costly to the public (Hyman 2007).

   The FDA, for instance, may face criticism for delaying a drug's approval, but that is nothing compared to the consequences of approving a drug that turns out to be unsafe. Frances Kelsey, an FDA scientist, stubbornly blocked the approval of thalidomide, which was eventually shown to cause birth defects; John F. Kennedy presented her with the President's Award. No FDA official was ever so honored for approving a breakthrough drug. For the FDA, fear of criticism thus—not irrationally—impedes work for the public good, and promising medications are delayed by years of hypercompulsive testing.

© Springer International Publishing Switzerland 2016
S.N. Whitney, *Balanced Ethics Review*,
DOI 10.1007/978-3-319-20705-6_8

OHRP is in a similar bind. It seems not to dream that it might play a positive role in improving public health and reducing health disparities, and I have never heard OHRP praised for supporting an IRB when it found a way to help lifesaving research proceed. Instead, OHRP is castigated when it reprimands fewer IRBs this year than last (Big Drop in OHRP Letters 2011). Both agencies will be cautious to a fault so long as society blames them for their errors and takes their successes for granted.

Their wary attitude extends to your IRB.

8.2   Your IRB and the Agencies

In the 1960s, the typical IRB had borrowed staff, paltry status, and no incentive to protect its institutional future. It was therefore in an ideally objective position with regard to scientists who might have a conflict of interest. Over the next 30 years, IRBs grew modestly, with most acquiring permanent space and staff, but remained out of the spotlight. Their relationship with the FDA and the Office for Protection from Research Risks (OPRR—OHRP's predecessor) was for the most part collaborative.

The end was abrupt. Beginning in 1998, OPRR temporarily shut down federally funded research at about a dozen major research institutions; the FDA joined in three of the suspensions (Brainard 2000). The sudden halt of federally funded research was a heavy blow to these organizations' prestige, finances, and operations. There was nothing unique about the institutions that were punished; their IRBs were struggling to keep up with their workload, but so were many others.

These aggressive enforcement actions struck fear in other universities and medical schools, who realized they could be next (Brainard 2000; Rubin 2001). In response, both affected and unaffected institutions showered new money and manpower on their IRBs. These well-supported committees were in no doubt that government sanctions must be avoided at all costs.

8.2.1 Balancing Three Goals

The burst of disciplinary actions subsided in 2001, but the threat remains. In today's anxious atmosphere, your IRB must do more than protect subjects and permit research to be conducted; you must also avert federal sanctions and so protect the reputation of the institution, the funding of the investigator, the job of the IRB chair, and the livelihood of the administrator and staff. This third goal, which is of course nowhere to be found in the regulations, has led to some confusion; commentators sometimes note disapprovingly that IRBs act to protect their institutions, (Sieber and Levine 2004; Fost and Levine 2007; Davis and Hurley 2014, p. 10) but to forget the institution's welfare would be irresponsible.

Your duty to protect your institution from federal punishment is a central reality of contemporary research ethics. Your IRB must do all you can to be in full compliance with the regulations as the agencies interpret them.

You cannot avoid all risk. This manual provides general advice about what ethics suggests, but you should always bear regulatory reality in mind. Most IRBs err on the side of caution, and in today's unreasonable climate that sometimes makes sense. We can move to a better system only if the federal agencies are persuaded to be more reasonable; but I do not advise your IRB to be the agent of change. If you want to help, join in the academic and political struggle for reform that is underway.

8.2.2 When Regulations Trump Ethics

In theory, the FDA and OHRP could employ experts in ethics to review an IRB's decisions, but both agencies spurn ethical debate. Jerry Menikoff, before he became director of OHRP, noted that in the "extensive list of the significant noncompliance findings" that OHRP might make when it audits an IRB, "there is not a single mention of the Belmont Report" (Menikoff 2007). I believe that neither agency has ever criticized how an IRB weighed ethical principles.

Federal auditors focus instead on two matters that may appear to be objective:

- How carefully an IRB follows the regulations, and
- How scrupulously the IRB *documents* that it has followed the regulations.

Despite the federal agencies' absolutist posture, whether or not an IRB has complied with the regulations is often a matter of judgment. Reasonable people can disagree on what, for instance, constitutes adequate information regarding a study's risks and benefits, yet the agencies act as if these were matters of black and white. It's no wonder that IRBs fear a federal audit (Klitzman 2012b). Audits are not an everyday occurrence—the agencies' modest enforcement staffs oversee thousands of IRBs—but they do happen, and every IRB must be prepared.

While there may be dispute over ethical judgments, there is no disagreement on the need for careful documentation. If you meticulously follow, and document that you have followed, appropriate procedures, the federal auditors are more likely to be smiling as they finish their review of your records.

8.2.3   The Successful IRB

Most successful IRBs have a productive division of executive labor between two people, the chair and the administrator. The chair sets policy, runs the meetings, talks with investigators, and is the board's public voice. The chair, who uses the regulations to meet ethical goals, knows that the regulations provide for exceptions, like the IRB's authority to waive the customary requirement for consent. The chair keeps the IRB ethical.

Most successful IRBs have an administrator with a fetish for order. The administrator, who works closely with the chair, knows the regulations and the board's standing operating procedures, often better than the members do, and maintains records that prove that the IRB has faithfully performed its duties. The administrator keeps the IRB in compliance.

8.2.4 *Things Can Go Wrong*

American biomedical research is remarkably safe, but subjects can still be injured. When a research subject dies unexpectedly, one or both federal agencies are likely to conduct a searching audit. With the benefit of hindsight, they can usually determine that errors were made.

Fortunately, injuries are uncommon and fatalities are rare, with about five unexpected deaths out of many millions of research subjects in America in the last 15 years. Far more often, an agency disagrees with an IRB's decision even though no subject has been harmed; this is usually how an IRB finds itself in the federal crosshairs.

8.3 Pushing Back Against Federal Pressure

Let's assume—and I am hoping this never happens—that the FDA or OHRP believes that your IRB has erred. What are your options?

Most institutions, confronted with federal sanctions, roll belly-up into a submissive display. This may be more prudent than craven, but there are ways to resist should you choose to do so.

8.3.1 *The Agency*

You can ask the agency to reconsider. This should be done in writing and should be accompanied by any material that supports your case. Politely point out any errors in the agency's recitation of facts or analysis. Bring in additional documentation. Attach expert rebuttals.

If that fails, there are other possibilities. In our system of government, unfavorable agency actions can be challenged through scientific or political channels, the courts, and the media. A medical school under attack by OHRP can, for instance, look for help from the agency that felt its research was ethically sound when it funded it.

8.3.2   The Funder

The University of Alabama at Birmingham (UAB) was one of the lead institutions in the SUPPORT study of respiratory treatment of premature infants (see also Sects. 7.4.3 and 7.6.2). In March, 2013, OHRP determined that UAB had violated the regulations by using a consent form that did not adequately describe the risk of the oxygen the babies were given (Buchanan 2013a).

OHRP's determination would have made sense had the UAB form failed to describe the risks of a new and unproven treatment. But this was a comparative effectiveness trial, in which every infant received care that was given routinely outside of the trial. Doctors never sit down with the parents of a premature baby to ask for their consent to administer oxygen. It has known hazards, but the consent form described its risks with great care.

Many experts felt that OHRP's rationale was specious (Wilfond et al. 2013; Lantos 2013; Drazen et al. 2013; Magnus and Caplan 2013), but its pronouncement still carried the weight of federal authority. National media spread word of UAB's alleged deficiency, a major newspaper castigated an "ethical breakdown" (Editorial Board 2013), and a New Jersey law firm filed suit against the lead UAB investigator, the IRB chair, and the IRB members (Looney v. Moore 2013).

OHRP's action struck fear in medical centers across the country. As NIH later observed, "This controversy has alarmed some of the parents of infants who were in the study, confused the biomedical research community, and befuddled IRBs. Several other studies seeking new insights to improve care for these vulnerable infants have been put on hold as the field tries to understand the OHRP findings" (Hudson et al. 2013). John Lantos commented that "nobody knows, anymore, what is permitted, forbidden, required, or optional" (quoted in Defino 2014).

In ordinary circumstances, the best an isolated medical school in this circumstance could hope for would be that abject apologies and a substantial cash outlay would limit the disaster. But UAB was not alone; the SUPPORT study was a collaborative effort involving 18 highly respected institutions. The study was not minor; it addressed a fundamental problem in neonatology. And although prematurity is hazardous, the study, as a comparative effectiveness trial, added no risk.

In June, the NIH stepped in. Francis Collins, Director of the NIH, joined with two colleagues to state that "we respectfully disagree with the conclusions of the OHRP" (Hudson et al. 2013). OHRP still refused to drop its enforcement action, but did put it on hold (Buchanan 2013b).

This grudging response did not unwind all of UAB's troubles; the court case lived on and the public relations damage could not be undone. But the NIH intervention gave American IRBs and investigators hope.

8.3.3 The Media

Media pressure can also compel an agency to retreat. In 2004, Johns Hopkins intensivist Peter Pronovost and his colleagues found a remarkable new way to combat serious infections in hospitalized patients. These infections are caused by tubes that are inserted deep into the body's circulatory system—an ideal position to monitor body function, but also a dangerous point of entry for bacteria. Pronovost's team showed that requiring doctors to follow a specific checklist when inserting these tubes reduced potentially fatal infections to near zero, one of the most dramatic improvements in hospital care in memory (Berenholtz et al. 2004).

The subjects of the experiment, if there were subjects at all, were the doctors who were required to follow the checklist. The experiment succeeded because the doctors gave the care they should already have been giving so that the patients received care they should already have been receiving. Pronovost had found a way to make the doctors do their duty reliably.

Although this research saved lives, it was more an experiment in human engineering than in biomedicine; the Common rule was never meant to apply to an investigation of this kind. But OHRP declared that the Common Rule applied, that the research violated the rights of the human subjects, including the doctors, and that the study must be stopped immediately (Borror 2007).

The agency's action was greeted with incredulity. The most prominent critic was the surgeon and health researcher Atul Gawande, who wrote in a *New York Times* op-ed piece that OHRP is "in danger of putting ethics bureaucracy in the way of actual ethical medical care." Gawande's prescription was simple: "The agency should allow this research to continue unencumbered. If it won't, then Congress will have to" (Gawande 2007). OHRP, without admitting error, abruptly reversed its position (Office for Human 2008).

8.3.4   The Courts

Finally, federal agencies are subject to review by the courts. Challenges to actions by either the FDA or OHRP may be undertaken if the agency's action is arbitrary or capricious. An agency that attempts to regulate matters that are not properly within its jurisdiction may also be challenged (Evans 2014).

8.4   Risk and Your IRB

Your IRB's goal, of course, is to keep out of trouble. This is easier said than done (Klitzman 2012b), and some federal enforcement actions cannot be prevented. My hope is that you will continue your valuable work and not be paralyzed by fear. In the face of uncertainty, even caution offers imperfect protection from adverse federal action, and going beyond caution will imperil your other goals. Greg Koski, former chair of OHRP, cautions you against engaging in "reactive hyperprotectionism" that "can have a stifling effect on research productivity without meaningfully enhancing the safety and well-being of research participants" (Koski 2004).

Your IRB should not take careless chances, but if you seek perfect safety you will impose unconscionable costs on the research you supervise, the scientists who conduct it, and the public. Your IRB must itself accept a modicum of risk. Life is never free of hazard; not for the research subject, the scientist, or the IRB itself. It is only by accepting some risk that you can pursue your ethical goals.

Chapter 9
The Future

Your IRB's work will never be static. You will need to keep abreast of the growing evidence base about research ethics in practice and you may participate in reform of the system. I hope this manual gives you a secure ethical approach with which to meet these challenges.

9.1 Evidence

Your IRB should use published data in your deliberations whenever possible (Lantos 2007a). I encourage you to also contribute to our knowledge about optimal IRB functioning, by making your IRB itself (with appropriate notice and consent) a learning institution (Sieber and Tolich 2013, p. 207–212). This manual suggests a variety of opportunities; you can explore topics like these:

- How do investigators and IRB members experience your appeals process? Has it changed how you function? (see Sect. 3.1.5)
- Does your IRB protect scientists, research staff, or other third parties? If so, with what results? (see Sect. 3.2.1)
- What are the results when your IRB goes beyond the regulatory minimum? (see Sect. 3.2.3)
- How does your IRB use the literature reviews that scientists generate? Do the scientists find preparing them helpful? (see Sect. 4.2)
- Have you compared the scientific merit of protocols before and after your required modifications? (see Sect. 4.3.1)
- When do you decide that some research is without value? (see Sect. 4.3.2)

© Springer International Publishing Switzerland 2016
S.N. Whitney, *Balanced Ethics Review*,
DOI 10.1007/978-3-319-20705-6_9

- How does your IRB's view of the riskiness of specific protocols compare with that of potential or actual subjects? (see Sects. 4.4 and 4.5)
- Have you allowed investigators to obtain consent from prospective subjects for a study you have not yet approved? (see Sect. 4.6)
- What is your IRB's stance about overstating or understating risks and benefits in a consent form? What are the views of subjects and investigators in your institution? (see Sect. 5.3)
- If your IRB edits consent forms, have you compared the before and after versions for clarity and accuracy? (see Sect. 5.6)
- If your IRB decides that a particular protocol is too politically sensitive to permit, how do you reach that decision? (see Sects. 6.1 and 6.2)
- If your IRB modifies the wording of surveys and interviews, have you asked an outside expert to review the before and after versions? (see Sect. 6.5)
- Has your IRB found a way to show that your efforts to promote justice succeed? (see Sect. 7.5)
- How does your IRB deem subjects in a particular protocol to be vulnerable? What action do you take, and with what results? (see Sect. 7.6)

All are questions for which the extant literature is sparse. This research is responsive to the call of Ezekiel Emanuel and colleagues for "a data collection mechanism to evaluate the overall performance of the system, including how well IRBs are functioning and how research participants are being protected" (Emanuel et al. 2004). Others agree: we need more data (Gunsalus et al. 2007; Abbott and Grady 2011; McDonald et al. 2014).

9.2 Reform

This manual proposes that your IRB deliberately work to promote the welfare of both subject and society. If you are not already doing so, this in itself will be a kind of reform. Your work will also change for the better if you use evidence whenever possible and take advantage of the flexibility afforded to you by the regulations.

Institutional Reform. Change is also possible at the institutional level. The University of Michigan has been experimenting since 2007 with less-conservative interpretations of the regulations. For instance, it allows non-federally funded, low risk research to undergo continuing review every 2 years instead of annually (University of Michigan 2013).

Your university can go beyond this, since the federal regulations do not require IRB review of research that is not federally funded or supervised (Feeley 2007). The American Association of University Professors recommends that universities do exactly that, using separate tracks to review federally funded and non-federally funded research (American Association 2012). Note that state regulations may impose different requirements.

Intrainstitutional and Interinstitutional Collaboration. IRBs, institutions, and scientists have several options for working together to improve ethics review. The NIH, for instance, has established a central IRB to review cancer studies. Laura Stark has reviewed some models for sharing IRB decisions, including a private intrainstitutional decision repository at Sunnybrook Health Sciences Center in Toronto and a governmentally-funded repository in New Zealand that accepts information about IRB review and decisions from any country (Stark 2014, p. 182–183).

Changes in the Regulations. The regulations themselves need reform. In 2011, HHS and the Office of Science and Technology Policy proposed a variety of changes to the Common Rule (Office of the Secretary 2011). Scientists, professional associations, ethics scholars, and others submitted thousands of comments on the proposed changes.

The process is cautious, in part because the regulations are not HHS's alone; any alteration must be approved by the 16 other federal agencies and departments that share the Common Rule.

Changes in the Law. Even after the relevant agencies achieve consensus, they cannot change the regulations beyond the limits set by the relevant statutes, including the National Research Service Award Act of 1974. Only a change in the law will open the door for fundamental reform.

9.3   The Challenge

The IRB system has been challenged almost from the time of its birth. Scientists have been among its most insistent critics, and hundreds of investigators have documented their struggles to obtain timely and appropriate review. This manual is responsive to their concerns, and is intended, in part, to help you approve research where appropriate, but never without thought and care.

Take the time you need to fulfill your ethical responsibilities. You have a duty to permit sound research, but never at the price of lessened protection for subjects.

Dennis Mazur is concerned about senior institutional officials manipulating the IRB. He cautions that a research chief should not appoint IRB members who are committed to facilitating scientists' work, nor should the committee itself shift "from a committee dedicated to the protection of research participants to a committee dedicated to facilitating research" (Mazur 2007, p. 192).

Mazur is largely correct. Every IRB member should agree that subject protection cannot be left to investigators. In terms of its purpose, the IRB should not be dedicated to either goal at the expense of the other.

We return to the central theme of this manual. Ethics review that focuses solely on protecting subjects or facilitating research cannot reach sound conclusions. Time after time, on one protocol after another, your IRB must reach decisions that balance subject protection and our common need for the fruits of research. If you follow sound ethical and regulatory principles, use your experience, and trust your common sense, you will succeed.

References

Abbott L, Grady C. A systematic review of the empirical literature evaluating IRBs: what we know and what we still need to learn. J Empir Res Hum Res Ethics. 2011;6(1):3.

Advisory Committee on Human Radiation Experiments. Final report of the advisory committee on human radiation experiments. New York: Oxford University Press; 1996.

Amdur R. Evaluating study design and quality. In: Amdur R, Bankert EA, editors. Institutional review board member handbook. 3rd ed. Sudbury, MA: Jones and Bartlett; 2011. p. 91–5.

Amdur R, Bankert EA. Placebo-controlled trials. In: Amdur R, Bankert EA, editors. Institutional review board member handbook. 3rd ed. Sudbury, MA: Jones and Bartlett; 2011a. p. 171–6.

Amdur R, Bankert EA. The consent process and document. In: Amdur R, Bankert EA, editors. Institutional review board member handbook. 3rd ed. Sudbury, MA: Jones and Bartlett; 2011b. p. 53–8.

Amdur RJ, Bankert EA. Institutional review board member handbook. Sudbury, MA: Jones and Bartlett; 2011c.

American Association of University Professors, Committee A on Academic Freedom and Tenure. Regulation of Research on Human Subjects: Academic Freedom and the Institutional Review Board. 2012. http://www.aaup.org/report/research-human-subjects-academic-freedom-and-institutional-review-board. Accessed March 1 2015.

American Sociological Association. American sociological association code of ethics. http://www.asanet.org/about/ethics.cfm (1999). Accessed June 8 2014.

Arkenau H, Olmos D, Ang JE, De Bono J, Judson I, Kaye S. Clinical outcome and prognostic factors for patients treated within the context of a phase I study: the Royal Marsden Hospital experience. Br J Cancer. 2008;98(6):1029–33.

Armstrong R, Gelsthorpe L, Crewe B. From paper ethics to real world research: supervising ethical reflexivity when taking risks in research with the 'Risky' (online version). In: Lumsden K, Winter A, editors. Reflexivity in criminological research: experiences with the powerful and the powerless. Basingstoke: Palgrave Macmillan; 2014.

Aronson E. Not by chance alone: my life as a social psychologist. New York: Basic Books; 2010.

Atanasov PD. Double risk aversion. (2010). http://Papers.Ssrn.Com/Sol3/Papers. Cfm?abstract_id=1682569.

Baron J. Against bioethics. Cambridge, MA: MIT Press; 2006.

Baron J. Some fallacies of human-subjects protection, and some solutions. Cortex. 2015;65:246–54.

Baumrind D. Some thoughts on ethics of research: after reading Milgram's "behavioral study of obedience". Am Psychol. 1964;19(6):421.

Beauchamp TL. Autonomy and consent. In: Miller FG, Wertheimer A, editors. The ethics of consent: theory and practice. New York, NY: Oxford University Press; 2010. p. 55–78.

Becker HS. Sociological work: method and substance. New Brunswick, NJ: Transaction Books; 1970.

Beecher HK. Ethics and clinical research. N Engl J Med. 1966;274:1355–60.

Ben-Shahar O, Schneider CE. More than you wanted to know: the failure of mandated disclosure. Princeton, NJ: Princeton University Press; 2014.

Berenholtz SM, Pronovost PJ, Lipsett PA, Hobson D, Earsing K, Farley JE, et al. Eliminating catheter-related bloodstream infections in the intensive care unit. Crit Care Med. 2004;32(10):2014–20.

Berrett D. IRB overreach? Inside Higher Education. https://www.insidehighered. com/news/2011/03/18/brown_professor_sues_university_for_barring_her_ from_using_her_research (18 Mar 2011).

Big Drop in OHRP Letters, Open Cases Raise Questions of Agency Commitment. Report on research compliance. 2011;8(3).

Borror KC. Division of Compliance Oversight, OHRP. Letter to Daniel E. Ford, Vice Dean for Clinical Investigation. Johns Hopkins, July 19, 2007.

Brainard J. Spate of suspensions of academic research spurs questions about federal strategy: a U.S. agency, its own future uncertain, unsettles college officials with its crackdown. Chron High Educ. 2000;96(22):A29–30. A32.

Brendel DH, Miller FG. A plea for pragmatism in clinical research ethics. Am J Bioeth. 2008;8(4):24–31.

Brody BA. Research on the vulnerable sick. In: Kahn JP, Mastroianni AC, Sugarman J, editors. Beyond consent: seeking justice in research. New York: Oxford University Press; 1998. p. 32–46.

Buchanan LR. Division of Compliance Oversight, OHRP. Letter to Richard B. Marchase, V.P. for Research and Development, University of Alabama at Birmingham, March 7, 2013a.

Buchanan LR. Division of Compliance Oversight, OHRP. Letter to Richard B. Marchase, University of Alabama at Birmingham, June 4, 2013b.

Burman W, Breese P, Weis S, Bock N, Bernardo J, Vernon A, et al. The effects of local review on informed consent documents from a multicenter clinical trials consortium. Control Clin Trials. 2003;24(3):245–55.

Calabresi G. Reflections on medical experimentation in humans. Daedalus. 1969;98:387–405.

Calvey D. The art and politics of covert research: doing situated ethics in the field. Sociology. 2008;42(5):905–18.

Candilis PJ, Lidz CW. Advances in informed consent research. In: Miller FG, Wertheimer A, editors. The ethics of consent: theory and practice. Oxford: Oxford University Press; 2010. p. 329–46.

Capron AM. Subjects, participants, and partners: what are the implications for research as the role of informed consent evolves? In: Cohen IG, Lynch HF, editors. Human subjects research regulation: perspectives on the future. Cambridge, MA: MIT Press; 2014. p. 143–56.

Carlson EB, Newman E, Daniels JW, Armstrong J, Roth D, Loewenstein R. Distress in response to and perceived usefulness of trauma research interviews. J Trauma Dissociation. 2003;4(2):131–42.

Ceci SJ, Peters D, Plotkin J. Human subjects review, personal values, and the regulation of social science research. Am Psychol. 1985;40(9):994.

Chadwick R, Berg K. Solidarity and equity: new ethical frameworks for genetic databases. Nat Rev Genet. 2001;2(4):318–21.

Chalmers I. Regulation of therapeutic research is compromising the interests of patients. Int J Pharm Med. 2007;21(6):395.

Cohen J. HRPP blog. 2010. http://hrpp.blogspot.com. Accessed December 11 2010.

Cowan DH. Human experimentation: the review process in practice. Case West Reserve Law Rev. 1974;25:533–64.

Curran WJ. Governmental regulation of the use of human subjects in medical research: the approach of two federal agencies. Daedalus. 1969;98(2):542–94.

Davidson J. Covert research. In: Jupp V, editor. SAGE dictionary of social research methods. London: Sage; 2006. p. 48–9.

Davis AL, Hurley EA. Setting the stage: the past and present of human subjects research regulations. In: Cohen IG, Lynch HF, editors. Human subjects research regulation: perspectives on the future. Cambridge, MA: MIT Press; 2014. p. 9–26.

Defino T. With just one investigation in 2013, OHRP seems 'Invisible' after SUPPORT dust-up. Report on Research Compliance. 2014 (May).

Dickert N, Grady C. What's the price of a research subject? Approaches to payment for research participation. N Engl J Med. 1999;341(3):198–203.

Doll R, Peto R. Rights involve responsibilities for patients. BMJ. 2001;322(7288):730.

Drazen JM, Solomon CG, Greene MF. Informed consent and SUPPORT. N Engl J Med. 2013;368(20):1929–31.

Editorial Board. An ethical breakdown. New York Times. 2013 April 15.

The Editors. OHRP and standard-of-care research. N Engl J Med. 2014;371:2125–6.

Edwards P, Arango M, Balica L, Cottingham R, El-Sayed H, Farrell B, et al. Final results of MRC CRASH, a randomised placebo-controlled trial of intravenous corticosteroid in adults with head injury-outcomes at 6 months. Lancet. 2005;365(9475):1957–9.

Eisenberg L. The social imperatives of medical research. Science. 1977;198(4322): 1105–10.

Emanuel EJ, Wendler D, Grady C. What makes clinical research ethical? JAMA. 2000;283(20):2701–11.

Emanuel EJ, Wood A, Fleischman A, Bowen A, Getz KA, Grady C, et al. Oversight of human participants research: identifying problems to evaluate reform proposals. Ann Intern Med. 2004;141(4):282–91.

Epstein LC, Lasagna L. Obtaining informed consent: form or substance. Arch Intern Med. 1969;123(6):682.

Evans BJ. The limits of FDA's authority to regulate clinical research involving high-throughput DNA sequencing. Symposium: Emerging Issues and New Frontiers for FDA Regulation, Food and Drug Law Journal. 2014 October 20.

Faden RR, Beauchamp TL, Kass NE. Informed consent, comparative effectiveness, and learning health care. N Engl J Med. 2014;370:766–8.

Faden RR, Kass NE, Goodman SN, Pronovost P, Tunis S, Beauchamp TL. An ethics framework for a learning health care system: a departure from traditional research ethics and clinical ethics. Hastings Cent Rep. 2013;43(s1):S16–27.

Feeley MM. Legality, social research, and the challenge of institutional review boards. Law Soc Rev. 2007;41(4):757–76.

Fiscella K, Franks P, Gold MR, Clancy CM. Inequality in quality: addressing socioeconomic, racial, and ethnic disparities in health care. JAMA. 2000;283(19):2579–84.

Fitzgerald MH, Phillips PA, Yule E. The research ethics review process and ethics review narratives. Ethics Behav. 2006;16(4):377–95.

Fleischman A, Levine C, Eckenwiler L, Grady C, Hammerschmidt DE, Sugarman J. Dealing with the long-term social implications of research. Am J Bioeth. 2011;11(5):5–9.

Food and Drug Administration. Payment to research subjects—information sheet, guidance for institutional review boards and clinical investigators. 2014. http://www.fda.gov/regulatoryinformation/guidances/ucm126429.htm. Accessed July 22 2014.

Fost N. Consent as a barrier to research. N Engl J Med. 1979;300:1272–3.

Fost N. Waived consent for emergency research. Am J Law Med. 1998;24:163.

Fost N, Levine RJ. The dysregulation of human subjects research. JAMA. 2007;298(18):2196–8.

Frankel MS. The public health service guidelines governing research involving human subjects: an analysis of the policy-making process [PhD dissertation]. George Washington University; 1972.

Fried C. Medical experimentation: personal integrity and social policy. Amsterdam: North-Holland Publishing; 1974.

Galliher JF. The protection of human subjects: a reexamination of the professional code of ethics. Am Sociol. 1973;8:93–100.

Gawande A. A lifesaving checklist (Op-Ed). New York Times. 2007 December 30.

Getz KA. Clinical trial insights frustration with IRB bureaucracy & despotism. Appl Clin Trials. 2011;20(1):26–8.

Gordon BG, Brown J, Kratochvil C, Prentice ED, Amdur R. Paying research subjects. In: Amdur R, Bankert EA, editors. Institutional review board member handbook. 3rd ed. Sudbury, MA: Jones and Bartlett; 2011. p. 119–24.

Gostin LO, Hodge Jr JG. Personal privacy and common goods: a framework for balancing under the national health information privacy rule. Minn Law Rev. 2001;86:1439–79.

Grady C. Payment of clinical research subjects. J Clin Invest. 2005;115(7): 1681–7.

Greene SM, Geiger AM, Harris EL, Altschuler A, Nekhlyudov L, Barton MB, et al. Impact of IRB requirements on a multicenter survey of prophylactic mastectomy outcomes. Ann Epidemiol. 2006;16(4):275–8.

Gubar S. Living with cancer: the new medicine. New York Times. 2014 June 26.

Gunsalus CK, Bruner EM, Burbules NC, Dash L, Finkin M, Goldberg JP, et al. The Illinois white paper: improving the system for protecting human subjects: counteracting IRB "Mission creep". Qual Inq. 2007;13(5):617–49.

Hadjistavropoulos T, Smythe WE. Elements of risk in qualitative research. Ethics Behav. 2001;11(2):163–74.

Halikas JA. v the University of Minnesota, United States District Court, District of Minnesota, Fourth Division, 4-94-CV-448 (1996).

Halpern S. Hybrid design, systemic rigidity: institutional dynamics in human research oversight. Regul Gov. 2008;2(1):85–102.

Hamburg M. Testimony before the Subcommittee on Health of the Committee on Ways and Means, House of Representatives. 106th Congress. 2000 February 17.

Hamburger P. Getting permission. Northwest Univ Law Rev. 2007;101(2):405–92.

Han C, Braybrooke J, Deplanque G, Taylor M, Mackintosh D, Kaur K, et al. Comparison of prognostic factors in patients in phase I trials of cytotoxic drugs vs new noncytotoxic agents. Br J Cancer. 2003;89(7):1166–71.

Hansson M. Do we need a wider view of autonomy in epidemiological research? BMJ. 2010;340(7757):1172–4.

Hansson MG, Simonsson B, Feltelius N, Forsberg JS, Hasford J. Medical registries represent vital patient interests and should not be dismantled by stricter regulation. Cancer Epidemiol. 2012;36:575–8.

Harris J. Scientific research is a moral duty. J Med Ethics. 2005;31(4):242–8.

Herbst A, Cole P, Norusis M, Welch W, Scully R. Epidemiologic aspects and factors related to survival in 384 registry cases of clear cell adenocarcinoma of the vagina and cervix. Am J Obstet Gynecol. 1979;135(7):876.

Herbst AL, Scully RE. Adenocarcinoma of the vagina in adolescence. A report of 7 cases including 6 clear-cell carcinomas (so-called mesonephromas). Cancer. 1970;25(4):745–57.

Herbst AL, Ulfelder H, Poskanzer DC. Adenocarcinoma of the vagina: association of maternal stilbestrol therapy with tumor appearance in young women. N Engl J Med. 1971;284(16):878–81.

Hochhauser M. Memory overload: the impossibility of informed consent. Appl Clin Trials. 2005;14(11):70.

Homan R. The ethics of covert methods. Br J Sociol. 1980;31(1):46–59.

Homan R. The ethics of social research. London; New York: Longman; 1991.

Horng S, Emanuel EJ, Wilfond B, Rackoff J, Martz K, Grady C. Descriptions of benefits and risks in consent forms for phase 1 oncology trials. N Engl J Med. 2002;347(26):2134–40.

Hudson KL, Guttmacher AE, Collins FS. In support of SUPPORT—a view from the NIH. N Engl J Med. 2013;368:2349–51.

Humphreys K, Trafton J, Wagner TH. The cost of institutional review board procedures in multicenter observational research. Ann Intern Med. 2003;139(1):77.

Hyman DA. Institutional review boards: is this the least worst we can do? Northwest Univ Law Rev. 2007;101(2):749–74.

Icenogle DL. IRBs, conflict and liability: will we see IRBs in court? or is it when? Clin Med Res. 2003;1(1):63–8.

Ingelfinger FJ. Informed (but uneducated) consent. N Engl J Med. 1972;287:465–6.

Institute of Medicine (IOM). The learning healthcare system: workshop summary. Washington, DC: National Academies Press; 2007.

Institute of Medicine (IOM). Beyond the HIPAA privacy rule: enhancing privacy, improving health through research. Washington, DC: National Academies Press; 2009.

Institute of Medicine (IOM). Best care at lower cost: the path to continuously learning health care in America. Washington, DC: National Academies Press; 2012.

Jonas H. Philosophical reflections on experimenting with human subjects. Daedalus. 1969;98(2):219–47.

Kalven Committee. Report on the university's role in political and social action. 1967. http://www.bilkent.edu.tr/kalvenreport.pdf. Accessed February 7 2015.

Kass NE, Faden RR, Goodman SN, Pronovost P, Tunis S, Beauchamp TL. The research-treatment distinction: a problematic approach for determining which activities should have ethical oversight. Hastings Cent Rep. 2013;43(s1):S4–15.

Kass NE, Natowicz MR, Hull SC, Faden RR, Plantinga L, Gostin LO, et al. The use of medical records in research: what do patients want? J Law Med Ethics. 2003;31(3):429–33.

Katz J. In case of emergency: no need for consent. Hastings Cent Rep. 1997;27(1):9.

Katz J. Toward a natural history of ethical censorship. Law Soc Rev. 2007;41(4):797–810.

Katz J, Capron AM, Glass E. Experimentation with human beings: the authority of the investigator, subject, professions, and state in the human experimentation process. New York: Russell Sage; 1972.

Khan ST, Kornetsky SZ. Overview of initial protocol review. In: Bankert EA, Amdur RJ, editors. Institutional review board: management and function. 2nd ed. Sudbury, MA: Jones & Bartlett; 2005. p. 119–25.

Klitzman RL. The myth of community differences as the cause of variations among IRBs. AJOB Prim Res. 2011a;2(2):24–33.

Klitzman RL. The ethics police?: IRBs' views concerning their power. PLoS One. 2011b;6(12):e28773.

Klitzman RL. Institutional review board community members: who are they, what do they do, and whom do they represent? Acad Med. 2012a;87(7):975–81.

Klitzman RL. Local IRBs vs. federal agencies: shifting dynamics, systems, and relationships. J Empir Res Hum Res Ethics. 2012b;7(3):50–62.

Klitzman RL. How IRBs view and make decisions about social risks. J Empir Res Hum Res Ethics. 2013;8(3):58–65.

Koski G. Ethics, science, and oversight of critical care research: the office for human research protections. Am J Respir Crit Care Med. 2004;169(9):982–6.

Langmuir AD. New environmental factor in congenital disease. N Engl J Med. 1971;284(16):912–3.

Lantos JD. The "inclusion benefit" in clinical trials. J Pediatr. 1999;134(2): 130–1.

Lantos JD. Should institutional review board decisions be evidence-based? Arch Pediatr Adolesc Med. 2007a;161(5):516–7.

Lantos JD. Research in wonderland: does "minimal risk" mean whatever an institutional review board says it means? Am J Bioeth. 2007b;7(3):11–2.

Lantos JD. SUPPORTing premature infants. Pediatrics. 2013;132(6):e1661–3.

Lantos JD, Spertus JA. The concept of risk in comparative-effectiveness research. N Engl J Med. 2014;371:2129–30.

Levine RJ. Ethics and regulation of clinical research. Baltimore, MD: Urban & Schwarzenberg; 1981.

Levine RJ. Ethics and regulation of clinical research. 2nd ed. Baltimore, MD: Urban & Schwarzenberg; 1986.

Levine RJ. Empirical research to evaluate ethics committees' burdensome and perhaps unproductive policies and practices: a proposal. J Empir Res Hum Res Ethics. 2006a;1(3):1–4.

Levine RJ. Reflections on chairing an institutional review board. In: Bankert EA, Amdur RJ, editors. Institutional review board: management and function. Burlington, MA: Jones & Bartlett Learning; 2006b. p. 61–3.

Lidz CW, Appelbaum PS, Grisso T, Renaud M. Therapeutic misconception and the appreciation of risks in clinical trials. Soc Sci Med. 2004;58(9):1689–97.

Lidz CW, Appelbaum PS, Meisel A. Two models of implementing informed consent. Arch Intern Med. 1988;148(6):1385.

Lindgren J, Murashko D, Ford MR. Foreword: Symposium on censorship and institutional review boards. Northwest Univ Law Rev. 2007;101(2):399.

Looney, Billy Ryan et al v. Sheila D. Moore, Ferdinant Urthaler, MD, Individual Members of the University of Alabama Institutional Review Board, and Waldemar A. Carlo, MD. District Court of Northern Alabama (2013).

Magnus D, Caplan AL. Risk, consent, and SUPPORT. N Engl J Med. 2013;368(20):1864–5.

Markman M. Further evidence of clinical benefit associated with participation in phase I oncology trials. Br J Cancer. 2008;98(6):1021–2.

Mathews T, MacDorman M. Infant mortality statistics from the 2007 period linked birth/infant death data set. Natl Vital Stat Rep. 2011;59(6):1–30.

Mazur DJ. Evaluating the science and ethics of research on humans: a guide for IRB members. Baltimore, MD: Johns Hopkins University Press; 2007.

McDonald M, Cox S, Townsend A. Toward human research protection that is evidence based and participant centered. In: Cohen IG, Lynch HF, editors. Human subjects research regulation: perspectives on the future. Cambridge, MA: MIT Press; 2014. p. 113–26.

Menikoff J, Richards EP. What the doctor didn't say: the hidden truth about medical research. Oxford: Oxford University Press; 2006.

Menikoff J. Where's the law? Uncovering the truth about IRBs and censorship. Northwest Univ Law Rev. 2007;101(2):791–800.

Meyer MN. Three challenges for risk-based (research) regulation: heterogeneity among regulated activities, regulator bias, and stakeholder heterogeneity. In: Cohen IG, Lynch HF, editors. Human subjects research regulation: perspectives on the future. Cambridge, MA: MIT Press; 2014. p. 313–26.

Milgram S. Behavioral study of obedience. J Abnorm Soc Psychol. 1963; 67(4):371.

Miller FG. Revisiting the Belmont Report: the ethical significance of the distinction between clinical research and medical care. APA Newslett Philos Med. 2006a;5:10–4.

Miller FG. Consent to clinical research. In: Miller FG, Wertheimer A, editors. The ethics of consent: theory and practice. Oxford: Oxford University Press; 2010. p. 375–404.

Miller FG, Wertheimer A. Preface to a theory of consent transactions: beyond valid consent. In: Miller FG, Wertheimer A, editors. The ethics of consent: theory and practice. Oxford: Oxford University Press; 2010. p. 79–105.

Miller M. Phase I oncology trials. In: Bankert EA, Amdur RJ, editors. Institutional review board: management and function. 2nd ed. Burlington, MA: Jones & Bartlett Learning; 2006b. p. 455–64.

Morahan PS, Yamagata H, McDade SA, Richman R, Francis R, Odhner VC. New challenges facing interinstitutional social science and educational program evaluation research at academic health centers: a case study from the ELAM program. Acad Med. 2006;81(6):527–34.

Moss J. If institutional review boards were declared unconstitutional, they would have to be reinvented. Northwest Univ Law Rev. 2007;101(2):801–8.

National Bioethics Advisory Commission. Ethical and policy issues in research involving human participants — volume I. report and recommendations of the national bioethics advisory commission. Bethesda, MD: National Bioethics Advisory Commission; 2001.

National Cancer Institute. Consent to participate in a clinical research study: Evaluation of the natural history and management of pancreatic lesions associated with Von Hippel-Lindau. On file with author; 2011.

National Commission for the Protection of Human Subjects of Biomedical and Behavioral Research. The Belmont Report: ethical principles and guidelines for the protection of human subjects of research. DHEW Publication No. (OS) 78-0012; 1978.

National Research Service Award Act of 1974.

Nelson DK. IRB member conflict of interest. In: Amdur R, Bankert EA, editors. Institutional review board member handbook. 3rd ed. Sudbury, MA: Jones and Bartlett; 2011. p. 103–13.

Newman E, Kaloupek DG. The risks and benefits of participating in trauma-focused research studies. J Trauma Stress. 2004;17(5):383–94.

Nuremberg code. http://www.hhs.gov/ohrp/archive/nurcode.html (1947). Accessed February 9 2015.

Office for Civil Rights, National Institutes of Health, Department of Health and Human Services. Frequently asked questions on the HIPAA privacy rule. 2007. http://privacyruleandresearch.nih.gov/faq.asp. Accessed November 22 2014.

Office for Human Research Protections, Department of Health and Human Services. Press Release: OHRP Concludes Case Regarding Johns Hopkins University Research on Hospital Infections: Encourages Continuance of Work to Reduce Incidence of Catheter-Related Infections; Offers New Guidance for Future Research. 2008 February 15.

Office for Human Research Protections, Department of Health and Human Services. 2014. Draft guidance on disclosing reasonably foreseeable risks in research evaluating standards of care. 2014. http://www.hhs.gov/ohrp/newsroom/rfc/comstdofcare.html. Accessed November 22 2014.

Office of the Secretary, HHS, and the Food and Drug Administration, HHS. Advanced notice of proposed rulemaking (ANPRM): Human subjects research protections: Enhancing protections for research subjects and reducing burden, delay, and ambiguity for investigators. 76 FR 44512-44531 (July 26, 2011).

Pager D. The mark of a criminal record. Am J Sociol. 2003;108(5):937–75.

Penslar RL. The institutional review board's role in editing the consent document. In: Bankert EA, Amdur RJ, editors. Institutional review board: management and function. 2nd ed. Burlington, MA: Jones & Bartlett; 2006. p. 199–201.

Pool IS. The new censorship of social science research. Public Interest. 1980;59:57–66.

Rajczi A. Making risk-benefit assessments of medical research protocols. J Law Med Ethics. 2004;32(2):338–48.

Ramsey P. The patient as person: explorations in medical ethics. New Haven: Yale University Press; 1970.

Ravina B, Deuel L, Siderowf A, Dorsey ER. Local institutional review board (IRB) review of a multicenter trial: local costs without local context. Ann Neurol. 2010;67(2):258–60.

Rawls J. A theory of justice. Cambridge: Belknap Press of Harvard University Press; 1999.

Rhodes R. Rethinking research ethics. Am J Bioeth. 2005;5(1):7–28.

Rhodes R. De minimis risk: a suggestion for a new category of research risk. In: Cohen IG, Lynch HF, editors. Human subjects research regulation: perspectives on the future. Cambridge, MA: MIT Press; 2014. p. 31–44.

Rich WD, Auten KJ, Gantz MG, Hale EC, Hensman AM, Newman NS, et al. Antenatal consent in the SUPPORT trial: challenges, costs, and representative enrollment. Pediatrics. 2010;126(1):e215–21.

Rich W, Finer NN, Gantz MG, Newman NS, Hensman AM, Hale EC, et al. Enrollment of extremely low birth weight infants in a clinical research study may not be representative. Pediatrics. 2012;129(3):480–4.

Rivera SM. Reconsidering privacy protections for human research. In: Cohen IG, Lynch HF, editors. Human subjects research regulation: perspectives on the future. Cambridge, MA: MIT Press; 2014. p. 251–64.

Rubin P. Time to cut regulations that protect only regulators. Nature. 2001;414:379.

Russell-Einhorn M, Ellis GB. Human subject protections in the United States: perspectives from the Office for Protection from Research Risks. J Biolaw Bus. 1998;1(2):36–8.

Saltman J. Housing discrimination: policy research, methods and results. Ann Am Acad Pol Soc Sci. 1979;441(1):186–96.

Saver RS. Medical research and intangible harm. Univ Cincinnati Law Rev. 2006;74:941–1012.

Schrag ZM. Ethical imperialism: institutional review boards and the social sciences, 1965–2009. Baltimore, MD: Johns Hopkins University Press; 2010.

Shamoo AE, Khin-Maung-Gyi FA. Ethics of the use of human subjects in research: practical guide. New York: Garland Science; 2002.

Sieber JE, Levine RJ. Informed consent and consent forms for research participants. Am Psychol Soc Observ. 2004;17:25–6.

Sieber JE, Tolich MB. Planning ethically responsible research. 2nd ed. Thousand Oaks, CA: Sage; 2013.

Smith T. Ethics in medical research: a handbook of good practice. Cambridge, UK; New York: Cambridge University Press; 1999.

Stark L. Morality in science: how research is evaluated in the age of human subjects regulation [PhD dissertation]. Princeton University; 2006

Stark L. Behind closed doors: IRBs and the making of ethical research. Chicago; London: The University of Chicago Press; 2012.

Stark L. IRBs and the problem of "local precedents". In: Cohen IG, Lynch HF, editors. Human subjects research regulation: perspectives on the future. Cambridge, MA: MIT Press; 2014. p. 173–86.

Tyson JE, Walsh M, D'Angio CT. Comparative effectiveness trials: generic misassumptions underlying the SUPPORT controversy. Pediatrics. 2014;134(4): 651–4.

Tyson J. Dubious distinctions between research and clinical practice using experimental therapies: have patients been well served? In: Goldworth A, editor. Ethics and perinatology. New York: Oxford University Press; 1995. p. 214–7.

University of Michigan. HRPP innovation & demonstration initiative. 2013. http://www.hrpp.umich.edu/initiative/index.html. Accessed May 31 2013.

Van den Hoonaard WC. Walking the tightrope: ethical issues for qualitative researchers. Toronto; Buffalo: University of Toronto Press; 2002.

Van den Hoonaard WC. The seduction of ethics: transforming the social sciences. Toronto; Buffalo (NY): University of Toronto Press; 2011.

Van den Hoonaard WC, editor. Ethics rupture. Toronto; Buffalo: University of Toronto Press; 2016.

Vist GE, Hagen KB, Devereaux PJ, Bryant D, Kristoffersen DT, Oxman AD. Outcomes of patients who participate in randomised controlled trials compared to similar patients receiving similar interventions who do not participate. Cochrane Database Syst Rev. 2007;2:MR000009.

Ward E, Jemal A, Cokkinides V, Singh GK, Cardinez C, Ghafoor A, et al. Cancer disparities by race/ethnicity and socioeconomic status. CA Cancer J Clin. 2004;54(2):78–93.

Weijer C. Research involving the vulnerable sick. Account Res. 1999;7(1):21–36.

Weijer C. The ethical analysis of risk. J Law Med Ethics. 2000;28(4):344–61.

Weijer C, Emanuel EJ. Ethics: protecting communities in biomedical research. Science. 2000;289(5482):1142–4.

Weijer C, Miller PB. When are research risks reasonable in relation to anticipated benefits? Nat Med. 2004;10(6):570–3.

Weinfurt KP, Seils DM, Tzeng JP, Compton KL, Sulmasy DP, Astrow AB, et al. Expectations of benefit in early-phase clinical trials: implications for assessing the adequacy of informed consent. Med Decis Making. 2008;28(4):575–81.

Weinstein J. Institutional review boards and the constitution. Northwest Univ Law Rev. 2007;101(2):493–562.

Wendler D, Miller FG. Assessing research risks systematically: the net risks test. J Med Ethics. 2007;33(8):481–6.

Wertheimer A. Rethinking the ethics of clinical research: widening the lens. New York: Oxford University Press; 2011.

Wertheimer A, Miller FG. Payment for research participation: a coercive offer? J Med Ethics. 2008;34(5):389–92.

Whitney SN. The python's embrace: clinical research regulation by institutional review boards. Pediatrics. 2012;129:576–8.

Whitney SN, McCullough LB, Fruge E, McGuire AL, Volk RJ. Beyond breaking bad news: the roles of hope and hopefulness. Cancer. 2008;113:442–5.

Wilfond BS, Magnus D, Antommaria AH, Appelbaum P, Aschner J, Barrington KJ, et al. The OHRP and SUPPORT. N Engl J Med. 2013;368:e36.

Wootton SH, Evans PW, Tyson JE. Unproven therapies in clinical research and practice: the necessity to change the regulatory paradigm. Pediatrics. 2013;132:599–601.

World Medical Association. Declaration of Helsinki—ethical principles for medical research involving human subjects. 2013. http://www.wma.net/en/30publications/10policies/b3/. Accessed February 9 2015.

Index

This index focuses on chapters 2 through 9, which contain the manual's substantive discussion.

A

Accountability in IRB process, 26
Administrators of IRBs, 102
Advanced Notice of Proposed
    Rulemaking, 109
Advisory Committee on Human
    Radiation Experiments, 41
Affirmative action, 58–59
African Americans. *See* Discrimination,
    racial, research in; Health
    disparities; Vulnerable groups
Agencies, federal. *See* Federal
    agencies; Food and Drug
    Administration (FDA); OHRP
Alabama, University of, at
    Birmingham, 104–105
Altruism, 40, 41, 44
Amdur, Robert, ix, 55
American Association of University
    Professors, 109
American Sociological Association's
    Code of Ethics, 67
Appeals from IRB ruling, 26
Archival research, 71–77
    effects of beta blockers, 79
    ethical considerations, 73–74
    HIPAA, 75–78
    limitations of, 80–81, 83
    privacy, 71–77

risk of, 73
subject duty to participate, 74
vaginal cancer, 76
Armstrong, Ruth, 28
Army. *See* Navy
Aronson, Elliot, 61, 62
Ashkenazi Jews, 29
Audits of IRBs, 101–103
Autonomy, 13, 39–45, 49–50, 73–74,
    90–93

B

Bankert, Elizabeth, ix, 55
Baron, Jonathan, 91, 96
Baumrind, Diana, 62
Beauchamp, Tom, 74
    comparative effectiveness
        trials, 84
    definition of coercion, 25
    research without consent, 84
Becker, Howard, 67
Beecher, Henry K., vii, 2, 13, 40, 78
    improbable consent, 40
    protection of the vulnerable, 89
    research as dangerous, 78
Belmont Report, 13
    autonomy, 13, 39–45, 49–50,
        73–74, 90–93

© Springer International Publishing Switzerland 2016   123
S.N. Whitney, *Balanced Ethics Review,*
DOI 10.1007/978-3-319-20705-6

Belmont Report (*cont.*)
    beneficence, 13, 39–45, 73–74
    benefits of research, 87
    federal audits disregard, 101–102
    hazardous research, 39–45
    justice, 13, 73–74, 86–88, 90–93
    research without consent, 73–74
    respect for persons, 13, 39–45,
        49–50, 73–74, 90–93
Beneficence, 13, 39–45, 73–74
Biomedical research. *See* Research,
    biomedical, approach to;
    Research, biomedical, topics
Blogger, free speech of, 59–60
Brody, Baruch, 89

C
Calabresi, Guido, 20
Cancer
    phase 1 trials, 96–98
    vaginal, 71–72, 76
Carlson, Eve, 64
Case Western Reserve, 21
Ceci, Stephen, 59
Censorship, 59–60
Chalkley, Donald, 38–39
Chalmers, Ian, 27, 38, 96
    emergency research, 96
    research without value, 38
Chemotherapy, 96–98
Chicago, University of, 58
Children. *See* SUPPORT trial;
    Vulnerable groups
Clarity in IRB process, 25
Clinical Center, NIH, 14–15, 90–91
Clinical Research Committee, NIH,
    14–15, 90–91
Coercion, 25, 88, 92
Collins, Francis, 105
Common Rule. *See* Federal regulations
Communities
    consultation with, 94–95
    protection by IRBs, 29
Companies, protection by IRBs, 29
Comparative effectiveness trials, 83–86
    ethics of, 84

    and federal policy, 85–86
    research without consent, 84–86
    SUPPORT, 85–86
Confidentiality, 71–78
Congress, US, 77, 80, 87, 106
Consent forms, 5–6, 47–56. *See also*
        Consent process; consent process
    computer generated, 52
    format, 53–55
    goals, 47
    imperfect but adequate, 50, 56
    multisite, 47–48
    vs process, 47
    readability, 53
    subject understanding, 50–52
Consent process, 5–6, 40, 41, 44–52, 49,
        50, 63. *See also* Consent forms
    before approval of research, 45
    cost of, 48, 86
    enrollment bias, 86
    vs. form, 47
    goals, 47
    as subject protection, 40–41
    subject understanding, 50–52
Constitution, US, 59–60
Covert field research, 65–67
Curse of power, viii, 3–4, 27–31, 35, 40
    archival research, 72–73
    biomedical protocol modification, 37
    exceeding the regulations, 30–31
    litigation prevention, 29–30
    pursuit of justice, 87–88
    review of humanities, 57
    scope of IRB authority, 28–29
    social sciences, 65
    vulnerable groups, 88–89

D
Davis, Amy, 30
Debriefing in social science, 61
Deception in social science, 61
Declaration of Helsinki, 38
Department of Health and Human
    Services (HHS), 18, 77, 109
Dickert, Neal, 93
Diethylstilbestrol (DES), 72

Discrimination in employment, 68–69
Discrimination in housing, 68–69
Discrimination, racial, research in,
    2, 68–69
    IRB chair attitudes, 29–30
    IRBs and, 59, 68–69
Doll, Richard, 74

E
Eisenberg, Leon, 25
Emanuel, Ezekiel
    protecting communities, 29
    research in IRB system, 108
    research without value, 38
    risk benefit analysis, 43
Emergency research, 93–96
    community consultation, 94–95
    criteria for approval, 94–95
    ethics of, 95–96
Employers, protection by IRBs, 29
Employment discrimination, 68–69
English, IRB review of, 57
Epstein, Lynn, 50
Ethics. See Research ethics
Ethnic minorities. See Discrimination,
        racial, research in; Health
        disparities; Vulnerable groups
Evidence
    developed by IRBs, 107–108
    in ethics review, 12

F
Faden, Ruth, 15, 41, 74, 85–86
    comparative effectiveness trials, 84
    duty to participate in research, 79
    fallible consent, 41
    research without consent, 84, 94–95
FDA. See Food and Drug
        Administration (FDA)
Federal agencies, 8, 10, 18, 99–106,
        101–103, 106, 109. See also
        Federal regulation; Food and
        Drug Administration (FDA);
        OHRP
    consent form readability, 54
    conservative view of consent, 41

    ethics, 101–102
    imperfect subject understanding,
        40
    inaction, 99–106
    IRB audits, 101–102
    IRB shutdowns of 1998-2001, 100
    IRBs resist, 103–106
    literature reviews, 35
    under pressure, 99–106
    spurred IRB growth, 99–100
Federal law, 40, 109
Federal policy
    limitations of, 68, 85–86
Federal regulations, 30
    archival research, 75–77
    controversial research, 58
    emergency research, 93–96
    flexibility of, 45
    IRB evaluation of risk and benefit,
        39, 42
    limitations of, viii–ix, 80, 88–89
    as minimum standard, 30–31
    multisite trials, 47–48
    origin of Common Rule, 18
    readability of consent forms, 53
    reform of, 108–109
    vulnerable groups, 88
Field research
    disciplinary disputes over, 66–67
    IRB review of, 66–67
    risk, 65–66
First Amendment, 59–60
Fitzgerald, Maureen, 26, 42
Fleischman, Alan, 59
Food and Drug Administration
        (FDA), 35, 50, 53, 80, 88, 92
        See also Federal agencies
    drug approval criteria, 94–95
    inaction of, 99–106
    oversight of IRBs, 10, 18, 99–106,
        100–103
    under pressure, 99–106
    requiring drug trials, 83
    revised regulations of 1991, 18
    subject payment, 93
Fost, Norman, 95
Freedom of speech, 59–60
Fried, Charles, 81

G
Gawande, Atul, 105–106
Genetics, interview about, 59–60
Gostin, Lawrence, 73
Grady, Christine
    research without value, 38
    risk benefit analysis, 43
    subject payment, 90, 93
Gubar, Susan, 98

H
Hamburger, Philip, 60
Hansson, Mats, 79
Harris, John, 79–80
Head injuries, 93–96
Health disparities, 14, 78, 86–90, 99
Health Insurance Portability and
    Accountability Act (HIPAA),
    73, 75–77
Hexamethonium, 35
HHS. *See* Department of Health and
    Human Services (HHS)
HIPAA. *See* Health Insurance
    Portability and Accountability
    Act (HIPAA)
History, IRB review of, 57
Hochhauser, Mark, 51
Hodge, James, 73
Homan, Roger, 67
Housing discrimination, 68–69
Humanities, IRB review of, 57
Hurley, Elisa, 30

I
Infants. *See* SUPPORT trial
Informed consent. *See* Consent forms;
    Consent process
Ingelfinger, Franz, 40
Institute of Bioethics at Johns
    Hopkins, 15
Institute of Medicine, 78
Institutional Review Board (IRB)
    appeals from rulings of, 26
    audits of, 101–102

conducting balanced review, 17,
    18, 109, 110
developing evidence, 12
and federal agencies, 100–106
future of, 107–110
as HIPAA Privacy Boards, 75–77
litigation prevention, 29–30, 68–69
objective, 33–34
power of, 26, 27
pressure on, 110
for profit, 11
protecting institutions, 29–30,
    57–58, 101–103
resisting federal sanctions, 103–106
at risk, 100, 101, 106
scope of authority, 28–29
successful management, 102
unbiased, 48–49
understanding of research, 34
Institutions
    IRBs protecting, 29–30, 57–58,
    101–103
Interview research. *See* Survey and
    interview research
Investigators. *See* Scientists
IRB. *See* Institutional Review Board
    (IRB)
IRB administrators, 102
IRB members, 18–21, 36, 39, 101,
    107, 110
    chairs, 102, 104
    colleagues of scientists, 23–24
    community members, 20–21
    compensation, 19
    influence, 11
    litigation, 4, 19–20, 29–30
    transparency, 24
IRB process, 3–4, 23–31
    accountability, 26
    appeals, 26
    clarity, 25
    curse of power, 27–31
    efficiency, 25
    judiciousness, 26
    openness, 24
    rationality, 27

respectfulness, 23–24
restraint, 27
transparency, 24
IRB system
    goals, 14–16
    history, 12–13
    reform, 108–109
    structure, 18
    triumph, 21

J

Jewish Chronic Disease Hospital, vii,
    12, 88–89
Johns Hopkins Institute of Bioethics, 15
Jonas, Hans, vii, 13, 15
Journalism *vs.* social science research,
    59–60
Judiciousness in IRB process, 26
Justice, 13, 81–82, 86–89
    governmental pursuit of, 87
    private pursuit of, 88
    subject payment, 90–93

K

Kaloupek, Danny, 64
Kalven, Harry, Jr., 58
Kass, Nancy, 74
    comparative effectiveness trials, 84
    duty to participate in research, 79
    research-practice interaction, 78
    research without consent, 84
Kelsey, Frances, 99
Khrushchev, Nikita, 93
Klitzman, Robert, 23
    IRB pursuit of justice, 87
    IRB use of intuition, 43
Koski, Greg, 106
Ku Klux Klan, 66–67

L

Lantos, John, 82, 85, 104
Lasagna, Louis, 50
Latinos, 89
Lawsuits. *See* Litigation

Learning health care system, 78–80
    definition, 78–80
    ethical considerations, 79–80
    privacy, 79
    subject duty to participate in, 79
    today's IRB and, 80
Levine, Robert J., 41
    and community member, 21
    editing consent forms, 55
    risk of research, 39
    subject autonomy, 39
Lidz, Charles, 81
Lindgren, James, 67
Literature reviews, 35–36
    by investigators, 35–36
    by IRBs, 36
    origin of requirement, 35
Litigation
    IRBs shielding institution from,
        29–30
    SUPPORT trial, 104–105
    threat to IRB members, 19–21
Local regulations, 18
Lotteries, 91–92

M

Markman, Maurie, 97
Mazur, Dennis
    approach to consent, 50
    editing consent forms, 55
    literature reviews, 36
    pressure on IRBs, 17, 110
    surveys, 63, 65
    variability of subject preferences, 39
Menikoff, Jerry
    approach to consent, 50
    cancer trial participants, 98
    danger of trial participation, 82
    federal agencies and ethics, 101
    reduction in unethical
        research, 21
    subject payment, 92, 93
Mentally disabled persons. *See*
    Vulnerable groups
Meyer, Michelle
    free subject choice, 44–45

Meyer, Michelle (*cont.*)
    IRBs as risk averse, 42
    risks of surveys, 63
    variability of subject preferences, 39
Michigan, University of, 109
Milgram, Stanley, 61–63
Miller, Franklin, 43, 51, 93
Miller, Paul, 43
Minorities. *See* Discrimination, racial,
        research in; Health disparities;
        Vulnerable groups
Mission creep. *See* Curse of power
Moss, Jonathan, 58
Muldoon, Robert David, 93
Multisite trials, 47–48

N
National Bioethics Advisory
        Commission (NBAC), 20
National Institutes of Health (NIH),
        14–15, 18, 90–93, 109
    backs SUPPORT trial, 104–105
    pursuing justice, 87
    research funder, 11
    and unethical research, 14
National Research Service Act of 1974, 40
    reform of, 108–109
Navy. *See* Army
NBAC. *See* National Bioethics
        Advisory Commission (NBAC)
Nelson, Daniel, 19
*New England Journal of
        Medicine,* 40, 85
Newman, Elena, 64
New Zealand review repository, 109
NIH. *See* National Institutes of Health
        (NIH)
NIH Clinical Center, 14–15, 90–91
NIH Clinical Research Committee,
        14–15, 90–91
NIH Council of Public
        Representatives, 87
Nixon, Richard, 93
Nonmaleficence, 13
Nonprofit organizations and justice, 88
Nonscientist IRB members, 20–21
Nuremberg Code, viii, 95

O
Office for Protection from Research
        Risks (OPRR), 100
Office of Science and Technology
        Policy, 109
OHRP. *See also* Federal agencies
    authority over social sciences, 57
    comparative effectiveness trials, 90
    inaction of, 99–106
    overseeing randomized trials, 81
    oversight of IRBs, 99–106
    under pressure, 99–106
    social impact of research, 58
Oxygen, in infants, 90, 104–105

P
Pager, Devah, 68
Participants. *See* Subjects
Payment of subjects, 90–93
Penslar, Robin, 53, 55
Peto, Richard, 74
Pharmaceutical companies
        and justice, 88
Phase 1 cancer trials, 96–98
    chance of benefit, 97
    subject hope, 97–98
    subject perspective, 98
PHS. *See* Public Health Service (PHS)
Polio vaccines, 13
Pool, Ithiel de Sola, 60
Poor. *See* Vulnerable groups
Pregnant women. *See* Vulnerable
        groups
Premature infants. *See* SUPPORT trial
Principal investigators. *See* Scientists
Prisoners. *See* Vulnerable groups
Privacy, 71–77
Pronovost, Peter, 105–106
Protected health information and
        HIPAA, 75
Psychology research, 57, 60–63
Public Health Service (PHS), 14–15

Q
Questionnaire research. *See* Survey
        and interview research

R

Race. *See* Discrimination, racial,
 research in; Health disparities;
 Vulnerable groups
Rajczi, Alex, 44–45
Ramsey, Paul, vii, 13
 consent form bias, 48–49, 51
 on reasonable choices, 51
 scientists' bias", 33–34
Randomized controlled trials, 80–83
 benefits of participation, 81–82
 definition, 80–81
 loss of personal care, 80–83
 nonphysical risks, 82–83
 risks inside *vs.* outside, 81–82
Rationality in IRB process, 27
Rawls, John, 86, 96
Readability of consent forms, 53
Reform
 of federal law, 26, 109
 of federal regulations, 109
 of IRB system, 108–109
Regulation, principles of, 17–18.
 See also Federal regulations
Regulations
 federal (*see* Federal regulations)
 local, 18
 state, 18, 24, 109
Research assistants, protection by
 IRBs, 28–29
Research, biomedical, approach to,
 4–5, 33–45
 approval, 39–45
 consent before approval, 45
 IRB modification of protocols, 37
 IRB objectivity, 33–34
 IRB understanding, 34
 literature reviews, 35–36
 multisite trials, 47–48
 participation as benefit, viii
 pharmaceutical research, 27–28, 88
 scientists' bias", 33–34
 trends in risk, 38
 unnecessary investigations, 27–28
Research, biomedical, approach
 tounnecessary investigations,
 27–28

Research, biomedical, topics, 7–9,
 71–98
 archival research, 71–78
 comparative effectiveness trials,
  83–86
 emergency research, 93–96
 health services research, 71–78
 justice, 86–88
 learning health care system, 78–80
 phase 1 cancer trials, 96–98
 randomized controlled trials,
  80–83
 studies without value, 37–38
 subject payment, 90–93
 vulnerable groups, 88–90
Research ethics, 1–3, 11–21
 balanced, vii–viii, 15–16, 30–31,
  110
 evidence in, 12
 evolving, viii–ix
 goals, 14–15
 hazardous research, 39–45
 Paul Ramsey, 33–34, 48–49, 51
 people as focus, 16–17
 principles, 13
 and regulation, 17–18
 subjects *versus* society, 15–17
 theory, 13–14, 16–17
 triumph of, 21
Research, social sciences, 6–7, 57–69
 controversial, 57–60
 debriefing, 61, 62
 discrimination, 29–30, 58–59,
  68–69
 field research, 65–67
 IRB authority over, 57
 vs. journalism, 59–60
 laboratory, 60–63
 Milgram's shock experiment, 61–63
 social impact, 58–59
 survey and interview, 59–60, 63–65
 threats to self-esteem, 61–63
Research without consent, 76–77, 81–82
 archival research, 71–78
 comparative effectiveness trials,
  83–86
 emergency research, 95–96

Respect for persons, 13, 39–45,
        49–50, 73, 81–82, 90–93
Respectfulness in IRB process, 23–24
Restraint in IRB process, 27
Rhodes, Rosamond, 16
    duty to participate in research, 79
    subject overprotection, 42
Rivera, Suzanne, 73
Robespierre, Maximilien, 93
Roche, Ellen, 35
Rubin, P., 26

S
Saver, Richard, 82
Scandals, 12
    Jewish Chronic Disease Hospital,
        vii, 12, 88–89
    Tuskegee syphilis study, vii, 12,
        86, 89
Schrag, Zachary, 57
Scientists
    biased, 33–34
    colleagues of IRB members, 23–24
    at IRB meetings, 24
    IRBs protecting, 28
    respect toward IRB, 23–24
    value of work, 16–17
Scope of IRB authority, 28–29
    communities, 29
    companies, 29
    research assistants, 28–29
    scientists, 28
    third parties, 28
Self-esteem, threats to, 60–63
Shannon, James, 14–15
Sieber, Joan
    censorship, 59–60
    controversial research, 58, 59
    ethics of field research, 67
    interview research, 64
    Milgram shock experiment,
        62–63
    open IRB meetings, 24
    protection of research staff, 28
    shock experiment, 62–63

Social science research. See
        Research, social science
Society vs. subjects, 15–17
Southam, Chester, 12, 34
Spertus, John, 85
Stark, Laura, 29, 30, 43
    ethics of dissertation, 66
    ethics review collaborations, 109
    interview of IRB chairs, 68–69
    observation of IRBs, 66
State regulations, 18, 24,109
State universities and censorship,
        59–60
Subjects
    called participants, ix
    duty to participate in research, 74,
        79, 80
    imperfect understanding of
        research, 50–52
    injury or death, 103
    payment, 90–93
    right to choose, 41–42, 44
    vs. society, 15–17
    variability of preferences, 39–40
Sunnybrook Health Sciences Center,
        109
SUPPORT trial, 104–105
    federal sanctions, 85–86, 90
Survey and interview research
    constitutional issues, 59–60
    IRBs modifying, 65
    risks, 63–64

T
Thalidomide, 99
Third parties, protection by IRB, 28
Tolich, Martin
    censorship, 59–60
    controversial research, 58
    ethics of field research, 67
    interview research, 64
    Milgram shock experiment, 62–63
    open IRB meetings, 24
    protection of research staff, 28
    shock experiment, 62–63

Transparency in IRB process, 24
Trials
    benefits of participation, 82–83
    caffeine for infants, 49–50
    cardiac arrhythmia, 83–84
    comparative effectiveness, 83–86
    emergency, 93–96
    phase 1 cancer, 96–98
    Pronovost infection study, 105–106
    randomized controlled, 80–83
    SUPPORT, 85–86, 90, 104–105
Tuskegee syphilis study, vii, 12, 86, 89
    and justice, 86
Tyson, Jon
    safety of controlled studies, 82

U
Unaffiliated IRB member, 20–21
Universities, role in society, 57–58
University of Alabama at
        Birmingham, 104–105
University of Chicago, 58
University of Michigan, 109

V
Vaginal cancer, 71–72, 76
van den Hoonaard, Will, 65

Veterans Affairs National Center for
        Post-traumatic Stress Disorder,
        64
Vulnerable groups, 88–90
    and health disparities, 89–90
    and justice, 86–88
    regulatory overprotection of,
        88–89
    and SUPPORT trial, 90

W
Weijer, Charles
    component analysis of risk, 43
    and protecting communities, 29
    vulnerable groups, 88
Weinfurt, Kevin, 98
Weinstein, James, 60
Wendler, David
    net risks test, 43
    research without value, 37–38
    risk benefit analysis, 44
Wertheimer, Alan, 16, 51–52
    subject payment, 93
Wootton, Susan, 95

Y
Yale University, 21, 61